Atlas of Radiographic Positioning

Normal Anatomy and Developmental Variants

SHARON A. JAEGER, B.S., D.C., D.A.C.B.R.
Diplomate, American Chiropractic Board of Radiology
Private Radiology and Clinical Practices
Canoga Park and North Hollywood, California

Post Graduate Faculty, Los Angeles College of Chiropratic
and Cleveland College of Chiropractic, California

Formerly, Assistant Professor, Los Angeles College
of Chiropractic; Chairman of Department of
Radiology, Cleveland College of Chiropractic, California

With a Foreword by Edward L. Mauer, D.C., D.A.C.B.R.

APPLETON & LANGE
Norwalk, Connecticut/San Mateo, California

0-8385-0113-3

Notice: The author(s) and publisher of this volume have taken care that the information and recommendations contained herein are accurate and compatible with the standards generally accepted at the time of publication.

Copyright © 1988 by Appleton & Lange
A Publishing Division of Prentice Hall

All rights reserved. This book, or any parts thereof, may not be used or reproduced in any manner without written permission. For information, address Appleton & Lange, 25 Van Zant Street, East Norwalk, Connecticut 06855.

88 89 90 91 92 / 10 9 8 7 6 5 4 3 2 1

Prentice-Hall of Australia, Pty. Ltd., Sydney
Prentice-Hall Canada, Inc.
Prentice-Hall Hispanoamericana, S.A., Mexico
Prentice-Hall of India Private Limited, New Delhi
Prentice-Hall International (UK) Limited, London
Prentice-Hall of Japan, Inc., Tokyo
Prentice-Hall of Southeast Asia (Pte.) Ltd., Singapore
Whitehall Books Ltd., Wellington, New Zealand
Editora Prentice-Hall do Brasil Ltda., Rio de Janeiro

Library of Congress Cataloging-in-Publication Data

Jaeger, Sharon A.
   Atlas of radiographic positioning: normal anatomy and developmental variants / Sharon A. Jaeger.
     p. cm.
   Includes bibliographies and index.
   ISBN 0-8385-0113-3
    1. Radiography, Medical—Positioning—Atlases. 2. Anatomy, Human—Atlases. I. Title
RC78.4.J34 1987
616.07′57—dc19   87-25395
                                                                         CIP

PRINTED IN THE UNITED STATES OF AMERICA

*To my parents for teaching me
to believe in myself
and
Frankie and Salem
who were always there*

Contents

Preface xi

Foreword xiii
Edward L. Maurer

Introduction xv

   Helpful Hints xv

   Tube Rating Charts xviii

   Screens xviii

1. RADIOGRAPHIC POSITIONING AND NORMAL ANATOMY

Cervical Spine 1
   Anteroposterior Lower Cervical (APLC) 2
   Anteroposterior Open Mouth (APOM, OMO) 6
   Lateral Cervical 8
      Neutral 8
      Flexion 12
      Extension 14

Anterior Cervical Obliques 16
   Supplemental 20
      Bilateral Pillar View 20
      Unilateral Pillar View 22
      Off-Lateral of the C-7–T-1 Area 24

Thoracic Spine 27
   Anteroposterior Thoracic 28
   Lateral Thoracic 32
      Side-Lying 36

Lumbar Spine 39
   Anteroposterior *40*
   Anteroposterior Lumbar *40*
   Lateral Lumbar *44*
   Anterior Lumbar Obliques *48*
   Posteroanterior Spot *52*
      L-5–S1 *52*
      Anteroposterior Spot *52*
      L-5–S-1 *52*
      Lateral Spot *56*

Full Spine 59
   Anteroposterior Full Spine (For Scoliosis Evaluation) *60*

Pelvis 63
   Anteroposterior Pelvis *64*

Hip 67
   Anteroposterior Spot Hip *68*
   Frog Lateral *72*

Sacrum 77
   Anteroposterior Sacrum *78*
   Lateral Sacrum *80*

Coccyx 83
   Anteroposterior Coccyx *84*
   Lateral Coccyx *86*
   Lateral Sacrum and Coccyx *88*

Knee 89
   Anteroposterior Knee *90*
   Posteroanterior Knee *92*
   Lateral Knee *96*
   Tunnel View *100*
   Tangential (Sunrise) *104*

Ankle 107
   Anteroposterior Ankle *108*
   Medial Oblique Ankle (Mortise View) *110*
   Lateral Ankle *112*

Foot 115
   Dorsoplantar Foot (AP) *116*
   Medial Oblique Foot *120*
   Lateral Foot *124*

Toes 127
   Dorsoplantar Toes (AP) *128*
   Oblique Toes *130*

Calcaneus 133
   Plantodorsal Calcaneus *134*
      Tangential *134*
   Lateral Calcaneus *136*

Shoulder 137
   External Rotation (AP) *138*
   Internal Rotation *138*
   Stress View (AP) *142*

Elbow 143
   Anteroposterior Elbow *144*
   Medial Oblique Elbow *148*
   Lateral Elbow *152*
   Tangential Elbow (Jones' View) *156*

Forearm 159
   Anteroposterior Forearm *160*
   Lateral Forearm *162*

Wrist 165
   Posteroanterior *166*
      Dorsopalmar *166*
   Oblique Wrist *170*
   Lateral Wrist *174*
   Supplemental *176*
      Radial and Ulnar Deviation Views *176*
   Carpal Tunnel View *178*

Hand 181
   Dorsopalmar Hand (PA) *182*
   Oblique Hand *186*
   Lateral Hand *190*

Fingers 191
   Finger Series *192*

Skull 195
   Caldwell's Projection *196*
   Anteroposterior Towne's *200*
   Lateral Skull *204*
   Axial View of Skull *208*
      Base-Vertex, Submento-Vertex *208*

Sinuses 213
   Caldwell's Projection *214*
   Posteroanterior Water's *214*
   Lateral Sinus *216*

Ribs 217
    Anterior or Posterior Complaints   *219*
    Oblique Ribs   *220*
    Tangential Ribs   *222*

Chest 225
    Posteroanterior Chest   *226*
    Lateral Chest   *230*
    Apical Lordotic   *234*
    Full Chest Lordotic   *234*

Abdomen 237
    Posteroanterior Abdomen   *238*
    Kidney, Ureter, Bladder (KUB)   *239*
    Optional Lateral Abdomen   *240*

Bibliography 241

2. DEVELOPMENTAL VARIANTS

Cervical Spine 243
    Block Vertebra (Failure of Segmentation)   *244*
    Klippel-Feil Syndrome   *252*
    Sprengel's Deformity   *254*
    Hemivertebra   *256*
    Spina Bifida   *257*
    Absent Pedicle   *261*
    Agenesis/Hypoplasia   *262*
    Odontoid Abnormalities   *264*
    Ossiculum Terminale Persistens   *268*
    Occipitalization   *269*
    Anomalous Articulations   *270*
    Paramastoid Process   *272*
    Intercalary Bones   *273*
    Anterior Tubercle   *274*
    Posterior Ponticle (Ponticulus Posticus)   *276*
    Nuchal Bones   *278*
    Physiological Calcification   *280*
    Long Styloid Processes   *282*
    Cervical Ribs   *284*

Ribs 289
    Pseudoarthrosis   *290*
    Intrathoracic   *291*
    Agenesis   *292*
    Ectopic   *292*
    Synostosis   *293*

Forked *294*
Costal Cartilage Calcification *295*

Clavicle 299
Rhomboid Fossae *300*
Medial Ends *301*
Foramen *302*

Thoracic Spine 303
Hahn's Fissures *304*
Hemivertebra *305*
Persistent Apophyses *306*
Dorsal Hemivertebra *307*

Chest 309
Pectus Excavatum (Funnel Chest) *310*
Pectus Carinatum (Pigeon Breast) *311*
Azygos (Azygous) Lobe *312*

Lumbar Spine 315
Spina Bifida Occulta *316*
Knife Clasp Deformity *322*
Transitional Segments *324*
Hemivertebra *330*
Butterfly Vertebra *333*
Failure of Segmentation *334*
Anomalous Articulations *338*
Asymmetrical Facets *340*
Tropism *341*
Hypoplasia/Agenesis *342*
Persistent Secondary Ossification Centers *344*
Limbus Bone *346*
Nuclear Impressions *348*
Iliolumbar Ligament Calcification *349*

Pelvis 350
Paraglenoid Fossae *352*
Os Acetabuli *354*
Persistent Growth Centers *355*
Ligament Calcification *355*
Phleboliths *356*

Upper Extremity 359
Radioulnar Synostosis *360*
Conoid Process *360*
Supracondylar Process *361*
Persistent Growth Center *362*

Lower Extremity 363
  Fabella *364*
  Os Trigonum *366*
  Bipartite Patella *367*

Bibliography 368

Glossary 371

Index 375

Preface

Accurate patient evaluation is the goal of every doctor. Radiographs are an important tool in this evaluation process. Appreciating the normal and the variations that are not due to a pathological process is essential. By understanding how to produce films that best allow one to use this device, we can successfully complete the evaluation process.

This text presents the preliminary and essential information for basic radiography. The positioning portion is presented step-by-step, utilizing pictures and drawings that will assist you in simplifying the maneuvers. This text will assist students as they begin their study of radiography as well as provide a quick reference to the practicing doctor.

Depicting the normal anatomy opposite the technique will illustrate the end product and help you decide which view will best present specific structures. By presenting various examples of the anomalies and supplementing the pictures with text, I have attempted to give some consensus of what has been found in the literature as to the relevance of the altered anatomy.

Because biomechanics is an integral part of our practice, knowing what conditions affect this within our patient's is critical. This text is not meant to be the single reference when you encounter one of the many anomalies of the skeletal system. Hopefully, it will spur one to examine the journals and other references in the search for answers to the many questions that arise when we deviate from the expected.

I must express my appreciation to the many doctors and friends that with or without knowing contributed to this text. Just to mention a few: James Antos, D.C., Mario Arroyo, D.C., Rand Baird, D.C., Andy Baum, D.C., Stuart Baumgard, M.D., Michael Buehler, D.C., Michael Casey, D.C., Cleveland College of Chiropractic, Joan Davis, D.C., Shirley Dundas, R.T., Lori

Fujikawa, Al and Cheryl High, Paul Hollis, Lois Rasmussen, Howard Player, Don Leonard, D.C., Los Angeles College of Chiropractic, Mellinger Chiropractic Office, National College of Chiropractic, Bernadette Nolan and Deborah Pate, D.C.

Special thanks to Ed Maurer, D.C., for all his time and "suggestions" and to Joseph Howe, D.C. for his inspiration and guidance.

Thank you Kari Salinas-Troeger for the endless hours you spent typing and re-typing the final manuscript and to your children for lending you to me. My special thanks to Judy Rubinstein, A.R.R.T., who spent endless hours toiling over this manuscript with me, working at the x-ray machine and helping to evaluate the various means of material presentation. Also, to Gabrielle Rubinstein, Judy's daughter, for being my model. The endless hours posing and re-posing were much appreciated. Also thanks to Debbie L. Allen, B.F.A., who did the illustrations.

Foreword

For many years the chiropractic profession has been concerned about radiation protection and safety, particularly as it relates to the patient. Emphasis has been given to quality assurance of film production, reliability, and readability. With this has come a marked awareness of all phases of radiologic technology and the performance of those professional and paraprofessional individuals engaged in this activity.

Patient preparation and positioning, along with appropriate selection of radiographic procedure, remains at the heart of quality radiograph production. The student and practitioner alike have a need for an appropriate original learning experience and must have available a concise text that will permit easy accessibility and reference for use in the clinical setting. Recognizing this need, Dr. Jaeger has succeeded in capturing the basic elements involved in radiologic technology and has succeeded in presenting these in a markedly lucid manner.

Based on vast experience in teaching, coupled with comments from students, Dr. Jaeger has complemented the text with a section on normal anatomical variants which dramatically enhances the overall usefulness of this text. While perhaps unusual to be found in a radiologic technology textbook, the addition of the normal variant section will provide ready access and assist in film identification. This will aid the paraprofessional from confusion oftentimes created by variations due to trauma, disease, or occult pathology. This awareness of normal variation may well enhance quick determination of clinically significant abnormality, but may also prevent the production of additional radiographs due to a lack of recognition of normal variation. This section will undoubtedly be found extraordinarily useful to both the professional and paraprofessional when reviewing the finished radiograph.

Dr. Sharon Jaeger's background includes undergraduate work at Western Michigan University, a Doctor of Chiropractic degree from the National College of Chiropractic, and a residency in radiology completed at the Los Angeles College of Chiropractic. At present she serves as a member of the American Chiropractic Board of Radiology, indeed a position of honor and trust. Having witnessed her development into an extremely talented teacher who truly listens to the student and his or her concerns, it came as no surprise that she has undertaken the production of this text. As the reader will soon experience, the mix of academic and intellectual expertise coupled with a distinct, pragmatic presentation will make this work not only easy to comprehend, but totally functional in any facility. We can only hope that future refinements and additions to the current body of literature in this area will again be enhanced by works from Dr. Jaeger.

Edward L. Maurer, D.C., D.A.C.B.R.
Executive Vice President
American Chiropractic Registry of
Radiologic Technologists

Introduction

HELPFUL HINTS

Patient Clothing Restrictions

Give the following instructions to the patient when taking films of the noted areas.

Skull. Remove all hairpins, wigs, dentures, necklaces, eyeglasses, contact lenses, earrings, and all clothing that may be in or near the area being x-rayed. If necessary, put on a gown.

Cervical Spine. Remove all hairpins, wigs, dentures, eyeglasses, necklaces, and earrings. Remove all clothing in or near the area being x-rayed. If necessary, put on a gown.

Thoracic Spine. Remove all necklaces and clothing (including brassiere) in the area being x-rayed. Have patient put on a gown. It is wise to have patient take off their shoes if the film is to be taken upright.

Lumbar Spine. Remove orthopedic supportive devices and clothing above and below the waist. Underwear may be left on as long as there are no metallic clips, etc. Have patient put on a gown. If the film is to be taken upright, have patient remove shoes. Proper gonad shielding should be used.

Pelvis and Hips. Remove all clothing in the area including underwear if restrictive or bearing metallic clips, etc. Have the patient put on a gown. Proper gonad shielding should be used, provided it does not obstruct visualization.

When x-raying the lumbar spine, pelvis, or abdomen the 10-day rule should be considered for females of reproductive potential. According to the NCRP 33 the least likely time to expose an embryo is the first 10 days after the onset of menses. If it is essential that films be taken of these areas to ensure proper diagnosis of a patient, be sure to use correct technique and factors (fast film/screen combinations, proper collimation and as much shielding as possible).

Extremities. Be sure to remove all jewelry in the area.

Positioning Aids

Foam rubber wedges and blocks can be used, be sure they have no metallic compounds in their composition. Many x-ray accessory companies have proper wedges available. Due to natural oils it is wise not to place foam rubber wedges under the patient's mouth or head. Sandbags can be used for immobilization of patient.

Patient Measurement. X-ray calipers are used to accurately measure through the thickest part being x-rayed. The exceptions to this are the AP lower cervical, APOM, and lateral lumbar. The APLC and APOM should be measured skin to skin below the chin. The lateral lumbar measurement should be taken at the waist and another at the hips. The median between these two measurements should be used unless there is a greater than 6 cm difference, at which point a lateral lumbar should be taken using the waist measurement and a lateral spot film using the hip measurement. For chest films, be sure to include patient's full inspiration in the measurement.

When the measurement comes out to a ½ cm measurement, use the next higher whole number. If the patient is lying on the table as in a lumbar oblique, take the arm of the caliper and switch it around so the base of the calipers can rest on the table and the other arm can be placed at the thickest part being x-rayed. This avoids shoving the caliper under the patient and avoids patient movement.

Breathing. All views except those with listed special breathing instructions are taken with the breathing suspended. Be sure your patient is still while performing an exposure. Motion is the greatest destroyer of detail.

Tube Tilt. Lowering the tube 1 inch for every 5 degrees of tube tilt does not change the SID (FFD), but rather helps to maintain the original SID (FFD). This is most important in any view with a tube tilt over 20 degrees.

When there is a tube tilt, be sure to line the cassette up at the proper level, taking into consideration the angle of the central ray.

Identification. The film blocker should be placed so that it is out of the area of the parts to be visualized. Proper identification should include the patient's name or code, the date the films are taken, and the facility where taken. The age of the patient or date of birth is also recommended. The side of the patient closest to the film should always be marked. The marker is usually placed on the outer margin of the cassette, as there is not a lot of clearance between the top of the cassette and the grid. By placing it on the outer margin there is less chance of it being misplaced and overlying any structures you are trying to visualize.

To avoid confusion when taking oblique films it is best to use LAO, RAO, LPO, or RPO markers designating the way the film was taken. The following lists designate what you will see on each oblique.

Cervical Spine

RAO—right foramina (the side closest to film); right marker only placed behind spinous processes
LAO—left foramina
RPO—left foramina (furthest from film); right marker only placed in front of spinous processes
LPO—right foramina

Lumbar Spine

RAO—left facets and pars interarticularis (side furthest from film); right sacroiliac articulation (side closest to film); right marker only placed behind spinous processes

LAO—right facets and pars interarticularis; left sacroiliac articulation

RPO—right facets and pars interarticularis (side closest to film); left sacroiliac articulation (side furthest from film); right marker only placed in front of spinous processes

LPO—left facets and pars interarticularis; right sacroiliac articulation

Compensation for Osteoporosis

These guidelines also apply to patients with known conditions producing osteopenia, such as disuse, severe anemias, and certain systemic diseases. Decrease the kVp by 6 to 10 for thoracic and lumbar spine films. These guidelines apply to most females over the age of 55 and most males over the age of 60.

Compensation for Very Muscular Bodies

Add 10 kVp for very muscular patients; for children decrease mAs by one-fourth; for overweight patient's (excessive adipose tissue) decrease the kVp by 6 to 10 and double the mAs.

TUBE RATING CHARTS

A tube rating chart is included with every x-ray machine. Always be sure to check the charts that apply to *your* machine. Two focal spots—one small and one large—are a part of the equipment. To determine your tube's limits you should follow your mA station line across until it bisects the kVp line. At this point, you can determine the maximum number of seconds you can operate safely.

On the charts on page xix you can see by the darkened lines that with the small focal spot you can operate safely at the 200 mA station at 90 kVp at the stations below ⅜ second.

With the large focal spot you can use the 200 mA station at 90 kVp safely at time stations under 6 seconds.

SCREENS

In the early 1970s rare earth screens were introduced but not until the 1980s did their use become common practice. The use of this type of screen can reduce the patient exposure an average

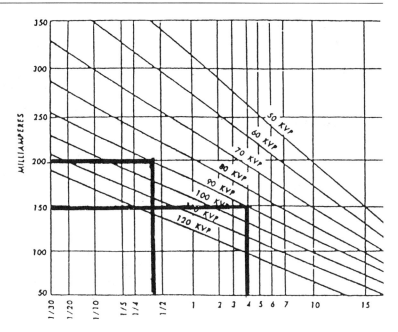

Maximum exposure in seconds: 1.0 mm small focal spot.

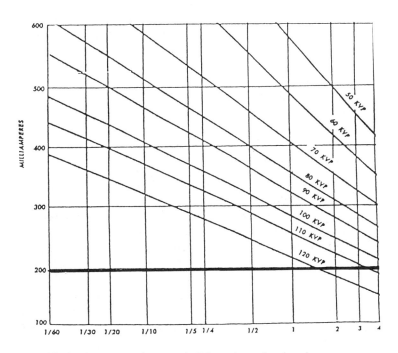

Maximum exposure in seconds: 2.0 mm large focal spot.

of 50 percent (averages of 33 percent to 92 percent mAs compared to conventional screens). The variations may be due to differences in installations, film/screen combinations, and body area being x-rayed. A decrease in kVp enhances contrast. When lower mA stations are used, the small focal spot can be utilized more frequently, thus providing greater detail. Detail is also increased when shorter times can be used minimizing the chances for motion. The reduction of the parameters should also increase the life of the x-ray tube. In offices with low powered equipment the use of rare earth screens can enhance the film quality and allow for more diagnostic x-rays.

Rare earth screens do, however, have some disadvantages—they are more expensive than hi-plus screens and the quantum mottle is greater, but these are not found to create significant alterations that diminish their diagnostic quality. The degree of permissable error is less. The life expectancy is 3 years rather than 5 years. However, with proper care this may be extended. Some rare earth systems may require a safelight change.

Film Screen Combinations

Combining the fastest film (800 system) with rare earth screens creates greater quantum mottle and compromises diagnostic quality. The 400 system (half speed) reduces patient dose significantly and will produce good quality films. The 400 system is less expensive than the 800 system. When hi-plus screens are used either the 800 or the 400 system can be used.

For extremities where greater detail is beneficial, the 200 system may be used or slower screens, such as detail or cardboard.

Cassette Screen Care

Clean and lint free screens help to provide clearer, better quality films. Periodically, you should clean your screens, especially when small particles or other artifacts (such as bugs, staples, etc.) are noted repeatedly on films.

Screens are best cleaned with a solution containing an antistatic compound and a mild detergent. Some liquid cleaners that may be used are

1. Commercial screen cleaner
2. Warm water and a very mild soap, such as Ivory liquid
3. *Pure grain* alcohol

The solution should be applied gently with a soft, lint-free cloth. *Never* rub vigorously. Never use your fingernails or a sharp object to remove particles. To dry, place the cassette on its edge like an open book. Be sure it is thoroughly dried before reloading.

Screens should be cleaned every 2 to 3 months unless it is a very busy office and then at least once a month. Cassettes should be stored in an upright position—never flat.

1
Radiographic Positioning and Normal Anatomy

Cervical Spine
Thoracic Spine
Lumbar Spine
Full Spine
Pelvis
Hip
Sacrum
Coccyx
Knee
Ankle
Foot
Toes
Calcaneus
Shoulder
Elbow
Forearm
Wrist
Hand
Fingers
Skull
Sinuses
Ribs
Chest
Abdomen

Cervical Spine

Anteroposterior Lower Cervical (APLC)
Anteroposterior Open Mouth (APOM, OMO)
Lateral Cervical
   Neutral
   Flexion
   Extension
Anterior Cervical Obliques
Supplemental
   Bilateral Pillar View
   Unilateral Pillar View
   Off-Lateral of the C-7 – T-1 Area

Anteroposterior Lower Cervical (APLC)

Grid
40″ SID (FFD)
15 degree cephalad tube tilt

70 kVp (optimum)
8 × 10 or 10 × 12 lengthwise

- Patient is supine or upright.
- The central ray is angled 15 degrees cephalad and enters 1 inch above the jugular notch (area of the thyroid cartilage). The head is tilted back slightly.
- Collimate to the angle of the jaw and laterally to a little less than film size. Measure skin to skin below the chin.
- Place the appropriate marker.
- Be sure to place the film in line with the angle of the central ray.

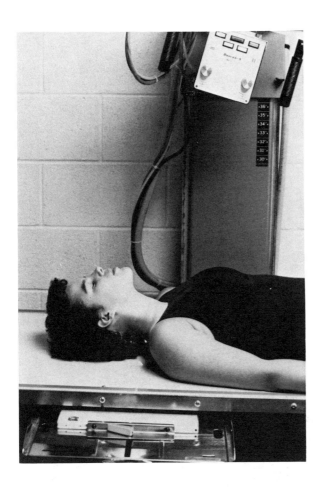

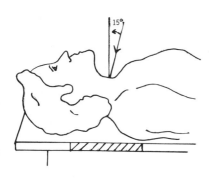

continued

Anteroposterior Lower Cervical (APLC)

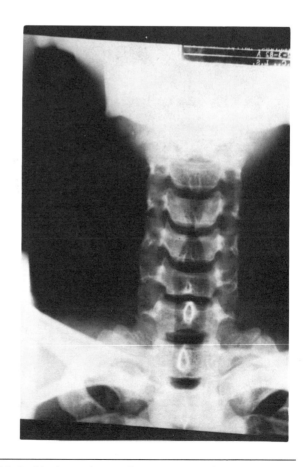

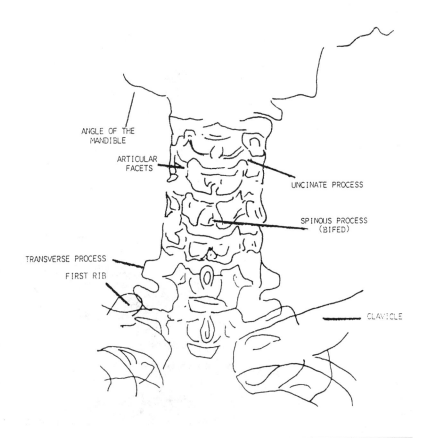

Anteroposterior Open Mouth (APOM, OMO)

Grid
40" SID (FFD)

70 kVp (optimum)
8 × 10 crosswise

- The patient is supine or sitting with mouth open as far as possible. The inferior borders of the upper incisors and the inferior border of the occiput should be in the same vertical plane. Sometimes it is necessary to have the patient bring his or her head forward a bit, (in the act of opening the mouth the head is thrown back). Be sure the head is not rotated.
- The central ray is at the uvula or even with the corners of the mouth.
- Collimate to just below the nose and laterally to the skin of the cheeks (approximately 3" × 5"). Measure skin to skin below the chin. Use the same factors as used for the APLC only double the mAs.
- Place the appropriate marker.

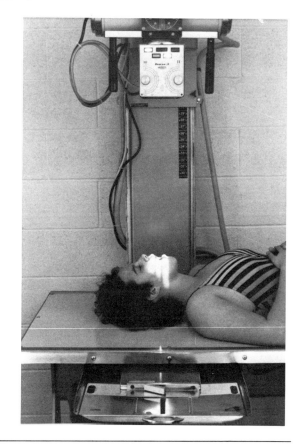

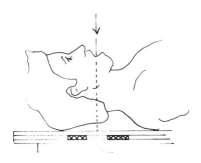

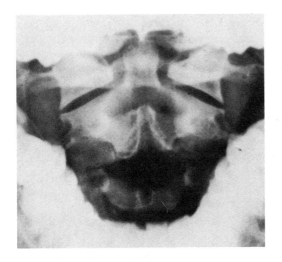

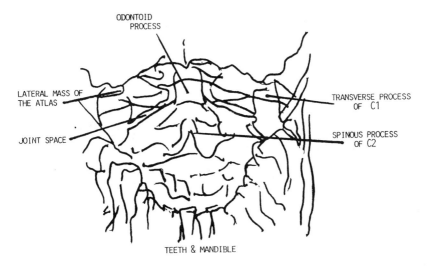

Anteroposterior Open Mouth (APOM, OMO)

Lateral Cervical

Neutral

Non-Grid (chest plate holder)   70 kVp (optimum)
72" SID (FFD)   10 × 12 or 8 × 10 film

- The patient is standing or seated with his or her shoulder touching the cassette and the head is parallel to the cassette.
- The central ray is at C-3.
- Collimate behind the eyes, being careful to include all the posterior structures and superiorly to 2 inches above the ear, being sure C-7 is included. Measure laterally skin to skin.
- Place an appropriate marker indicating the side closest to the film. Be sure the marker is not in the way of structures you wish to visualize. Sandbags may be held to bring the shoulders down in patients with thick, short necks.

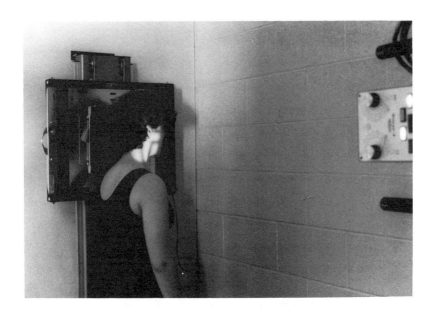

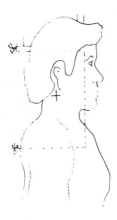

continued

Lateral Cervical: Neutral

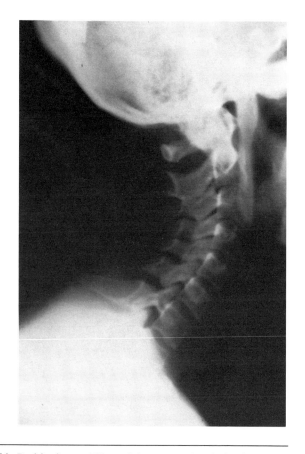

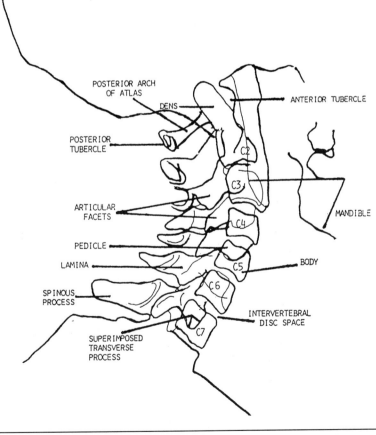

Flexion

Non-Grid (chest plate holder)
72" SID (FFD)

70 kVp (optimum)
8 × 10 or 10 × 12 film
Depending upon patient's ability to flex, it may be necessary to place the cassette crosswise.

- The patient is standing or seated with his or her shoulder touching the cassette. The head is parallel to the cassette. Have the patient (1) tuck his or her chin, then (2) flex the head and neck as far forward as possible (comfortably).
- The central ray is at the level of C-4 in the center of the neck.
- Collimate to behind the eyes, being sure to position the patient so you can still include all of the cervical vertebrae.
- Place the appropriate marker.

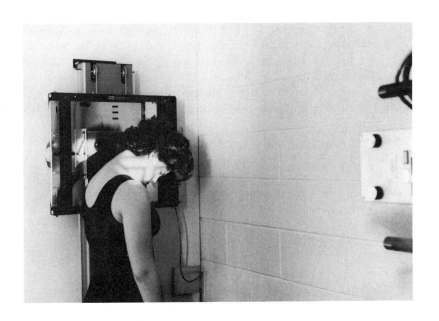

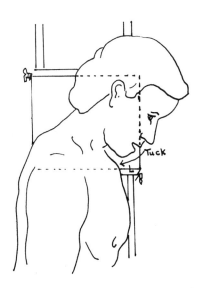

Lateral Cervical: Flexion 13

Extension

Non-Grid (chest plate holder) 70 kVp (optimum)
72″ SID (FFD) 8 × 10 film or 10 × 12 if neck is long

- The patient is standing or seated with his or her shoulder touching the cassette. The head is parallel to the cassette. Have the patient extend the head and neck as far back as possible (comfortably).
- The central ray is at C-3–C-4.
- Collimate behind or below the eyes.
- Place the appropriate marker indicating the side closest to the film.

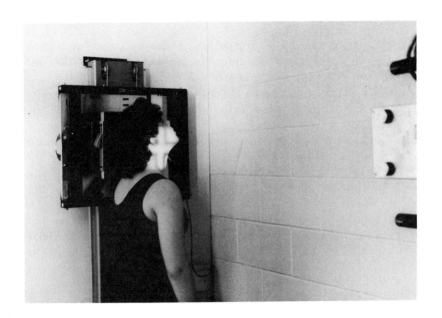

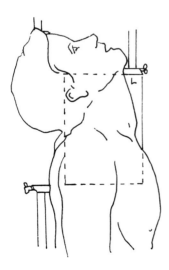

Lateral Cervical: Extension

Anterior Cervical Obliques

Non-Grid (chest plate holder)   70 kVp (optimum)
72" SID (FFD)   8 × 10
15 degree caudal tube tilt

- Patient is either standing or seated with their body at a 35 to 45 degree angle to the film. The head is parallel to the film, turned away from the anterior shoulder.
- The central ray is angled 15 degrees caudally and enters at C-2 or C-3 (approximately at the inferior aspect of the ear lobe).
- Collimate behind the eyes, being careful to position the patient so all the posterior structures are included. Collimate superiorly to the size of the film.
- Be sure to place the cassette on line with the angle of the central ray. This will place the cassette lower; the top of the cassette is often level with the superior margin of the ear. Measure laterally skin to skin (low about the C-6–C-7 level).
- Place the appropriate marker indicating the side closest to the film. The marker (*R* or *L* only) on the anterior obliques is always behind the spinous processes. The ID marker should be in an upper corner.

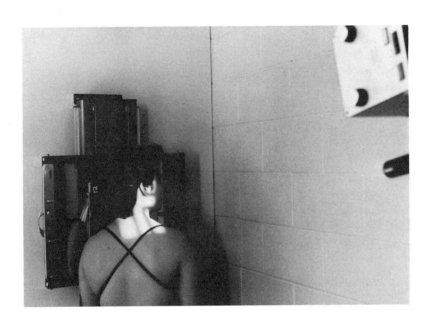

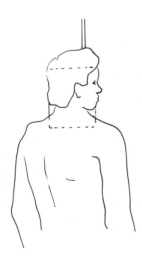

continued

Anterior Cervical Obliques

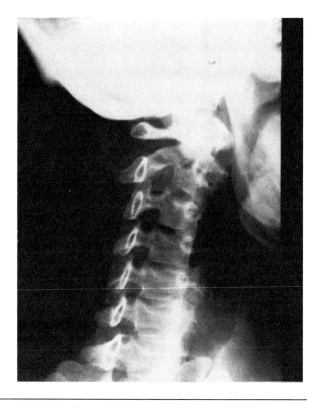

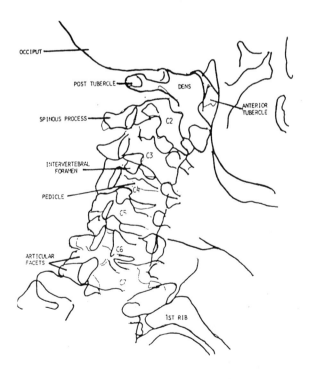

Anterior Cervical Obliques

Supplemental

Bilateral Pillar View

Vertebral Arch

Grid
40" SID (FFD)
25 degree caudal tube tilt

70 kVp (optimum)
8 × 10 film

- The patient is supine or upright (A to P) with the head hyperextended.
- Central ray is angled 25 degrees caudally and enters the neck in the region of the thyroid cartilage.
- Collimate to the lateral skin and to the chin superiorly.
- Measure through the angle of the central ray and place the cassette appropriately.
- Place the appropriate marker.

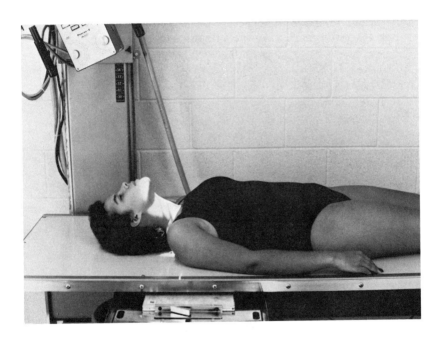

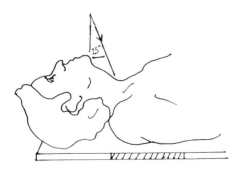

Supplemental: Bilateral Pillar View

Unilateral Pillar View

Grid
40″ SID (FFD)
30 to 35 degree caudal tube tilt

70 kVp (optimum)
10 × 12 film

- Patient is supine or upright (A to P) with head turned 45 degrees and slightly flexed.
- The central ray is angled 30 to 35 degrees caudally and directed toward the level of approximately C-4.
- Collimate laterally to skin, superiorly to film size.
- Measure through the angle of the central ray and place the cassette appropriately.
- Place the marker on the side opposite the face.

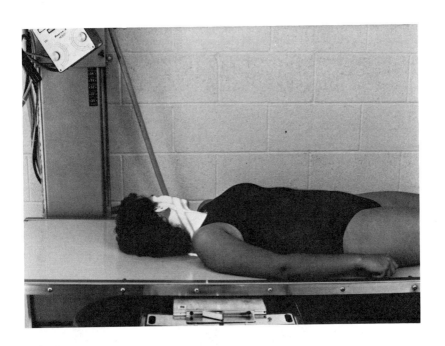

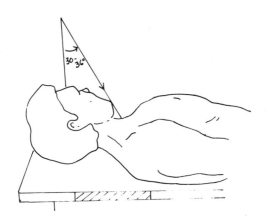

Supplemental: Unilateral Pillar View

Off-Lateral of the C-7–T-1 Area

Grid
40″ SID (FFD)
78 to 82 kVp (optimum)
8 × 10 film

- Place the patient in a lateral position, either standing or sitting then bring the shoulder closest to the film posterior and the opposite shoulder anterior raising the arm (somewhat like a swimmer's stroke). Do not rotate the patient. The head should be parallel to the film. The central ray is at the level of C-7.
- Collimate to a little less than film size.
- Measure through the central ray.
- Place the appropriate marker.

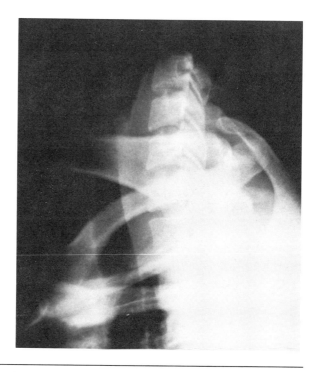

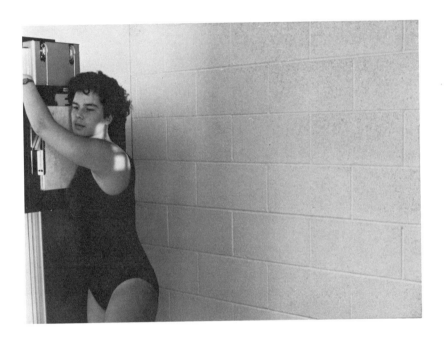

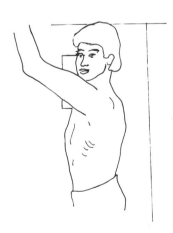

Supplemental: Off-Lateral of the C-7–T-1 Area

Thoracic Spine

Anteroposterior Thoracic
Lateral Thoracic
Side-Lying

Anteroposterior Thoracic

Grid
40" SID (FFD)

76 kVp (optimum)
14 × 17 lengthwise or 7 × 17

- The patient is either standing or supine. If the patient is standing, have him or her face the tube and step back to the grid until a body part touches. Have the patient distribute their weight evenly and put their hands down at their sides. (Be sure they are not rotated.) Place the cassette 1 inch above the level of C-7 or approximately 2 inches above the shoulder. If possible, filter the top one-third of the film or use the anode heel effect. The anode should be at the thinner part or toward the head in this case.
- The central ray is in the center of the cassette.
- Collimate to a little less than film size. Measure the patient over the shoulder, sternum to spine.
- Place the appropriate marker.
- The film is usually done on full inspiration to lower diaphragm.

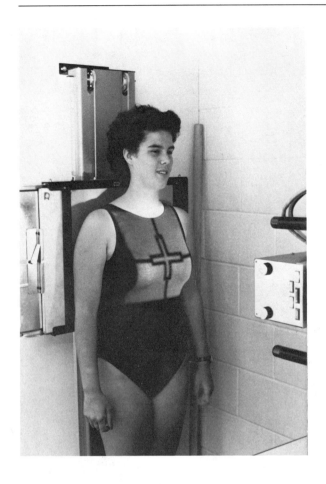

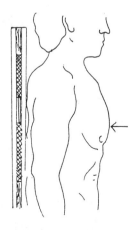

continued

Anteroposterior Thoracic

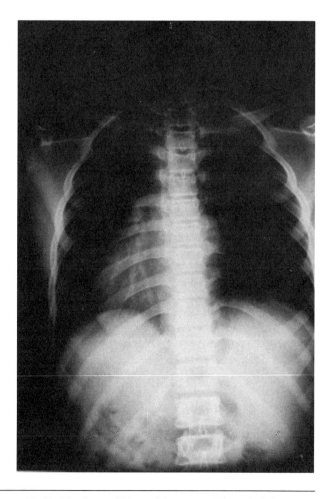

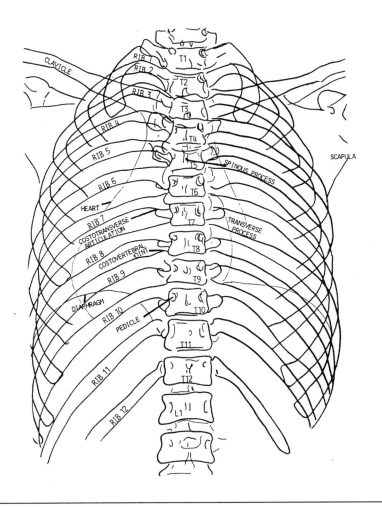

Anteroposterior Thoracic

Lateral Thoracic

Grid
40" SID (FFD)

80 kVp (optimum)
14 × 17 film

- Patient can be standing or seated. Have the patient roll their shoulders forward by crossing their arms in front them. Place the cassette 1 inch above C-7 or approximately 2 inches above the shoulders.
- The central ray is 2 to 3 inches in front of the spinous processes in the axillary region, at about the level of the sixth thoracic vertebra.
- Collimate laterally to the posterior skin and superiorly to the top of the cassette.
- If possible, filter the bottom half of the film or use the anode heel effect with the anode toward the lower thoracics.
- Place the appropriate marker.
- If the patient has a scoliosis, be sure to place the convex side closest to the film.
- Depending on the length of the exposure, to blur the ribs, you can have the patient employ rapid shallow breathing for an exposure of one-half second or longer. Be sure that the patient is not leaning against the grid.

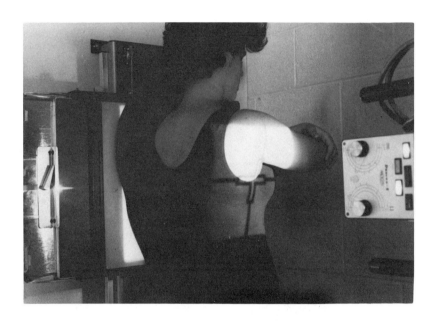

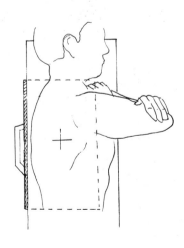

continued

Lateral Thoracic 33

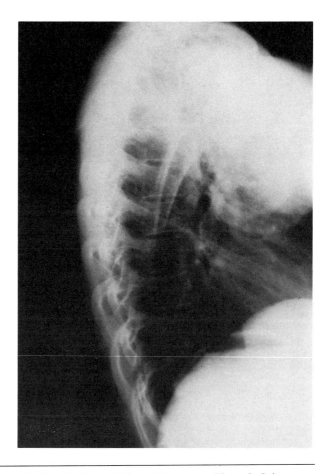

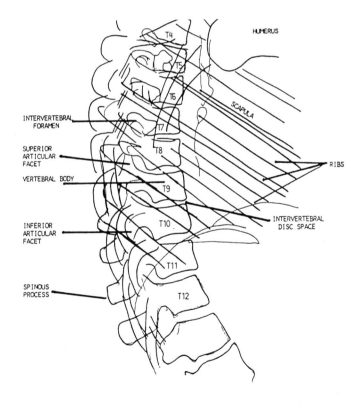

Lateral Thoracic

Side-Lying

Grid
40″ SID (FFD)
Approximately 10 degree cephalic tube tilt

80 kVp (optimum)
14 × 17

- The patient is side-lying. The mid-axillary plane is centered to the center of the table. The hips and knees are flexed to help support the patient. The patient's arms are raised so they are out of the way.
- The central ray is angled 10 degrees cephalad and enters at about the level of the sixth thoracic vertebra. If possible, filter the bottom half of the film or use the anode heel effect with the anode at the lower thoracic area. Measure through the axillary region.
- Collimate laterally to the posterior skin and superiorly to film size.
- Place the appropriate marker.
- This view is performed with respiration suspended.
- If the patient has a scoliosis, the side of the convexity should be closest to the film.

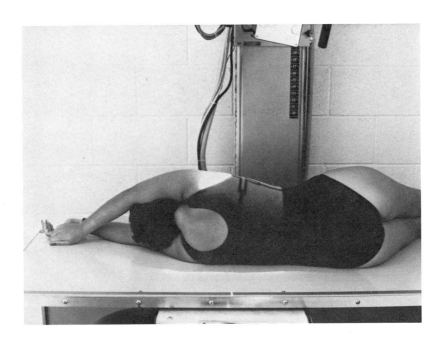

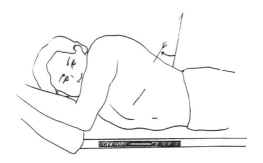

Lateral Thoracic: Side-Lying

Lumbar Spine

Anteroposterior
Anteroposterior Lumbar
Lateral Lumbar
Anterior Lumbar Obliques
Posteroanterior Spot
  L-5–S-1
Anteroposterior Spot
  L-5–S-1
Lateral Spot

Anteroposterior

Grid
40″ SID (FFD)

80 kVp (optimum)
14 × 17 film

- The patient is standing or lying with hands at sides.
- The central ray is at the top of the iliac crest.
- The symphysis pubis should be included. This is usually even with the level of the wrist.
- Collimate to a little less than film size.
- Measure through the central ray.
- Place the appropriate marker.
- If the patient is obese, the film may be taken PA on the table. This usually decreases the measurement, since the abdomen flattens out.

Anteroposterior Lumbar

Grid
40″ SID (FFD)

80 kVp (optimum)
10 × 12 or 11 × 14 film size

- Patient is standing or lying with arms at sides. Be sure the patient is not rotated.
- The central ray is at approximately the L-3 level.
- Collimate to a little less than film size.
- Measure through the central ray.
- Place the appropriate marker.

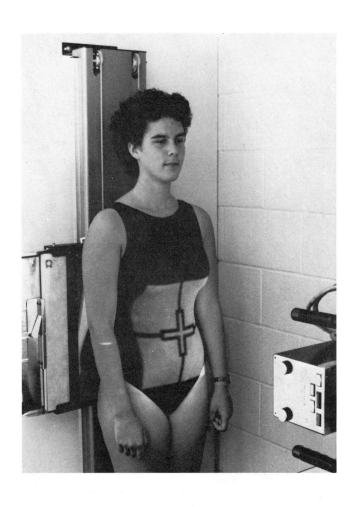

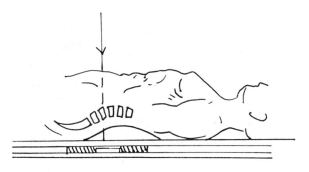

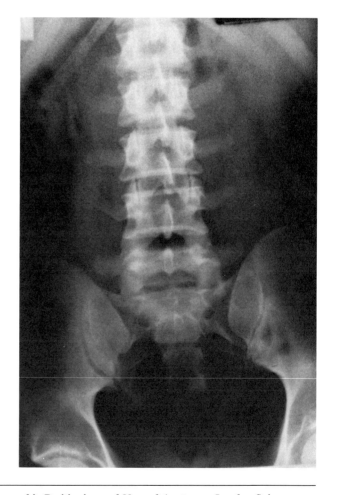

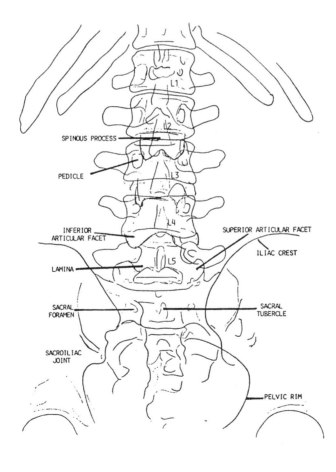

Lateral Lumbar

Grid
40" SID (FFD)

90 kVp (optimum)
11 × 14 or 14 × 17

- The patient is standing or lying 90 degrees to the grid with hands resting on the shoulders. If there is a large difference between the patient's shoulder and hip, it may be wise to wedge the smaller area to avoid movement.
- The central ray is about 1 inch above the crest and half-way between the ASIS and PSIS. Measure through the central ray. When measuring the patient, measure the hips and waist, and average the two. If there is a large discrepancy, 6 cm or more, take the measurement at the central ray and do a lateral spot film, if necessary.
- Collimate laterally to the posterior skin and superiorly to film size.
- Place the appropriate marker indicating the side closest to the film.
- If the patient has a scoliosis, place the convexity of the scoliosis toward the grid.

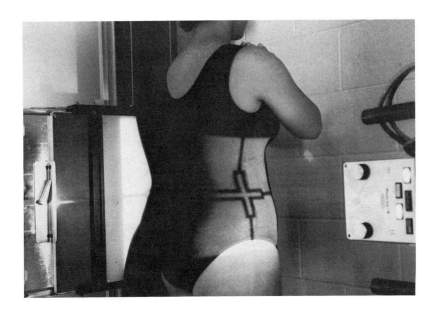

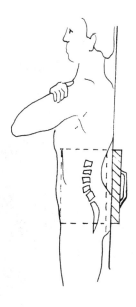

continued

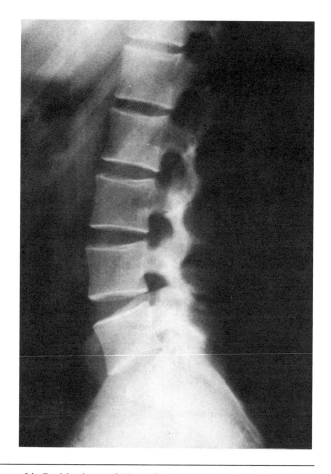

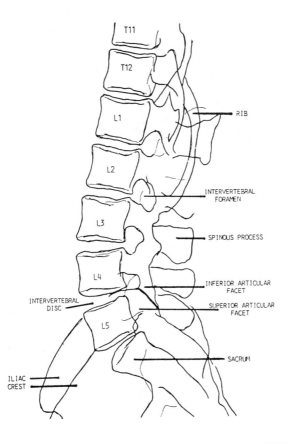

Lateral Lumbar

Anterior Lumbar Obliques

Grid
40" SID (FFD)

84 to 86 kVp (optimum)
10 × 12 or 11 × 14

- The patient is prone or standing (PA) with the body rotated approximately 35 to 40 degrees from the grid or tube. Place the arm closest to the grid down along the side of the body, raise the other arm toward the head.
- If the patient is recumbent the foot may be placed in the popliteal fossa for stabilization.
- The vertical central ray is about 1 inch superior to the spinous process at the level of L-3.
- Collimate to the length of the film and to 1 inch below the spinous processes (8 to 9 inches wide laterally). Measure through the central ray.
- Place the appropriate marker indicating the side closest to the film. The marker (*R* or *L* only) is always placed behind the spinous processes in anterior obliques.

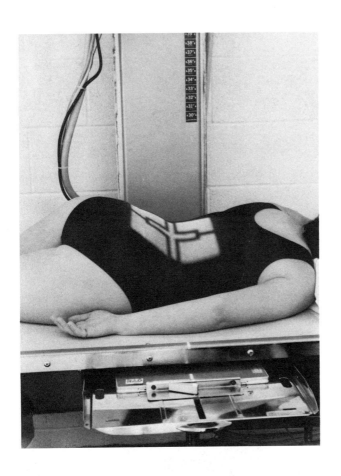

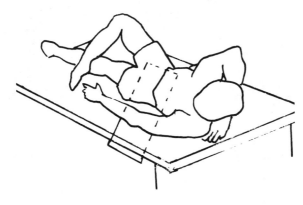

continued

Anterior Lumbar Obliques

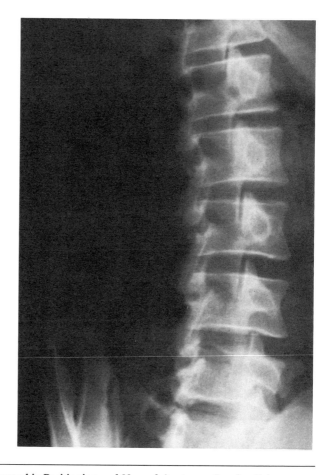

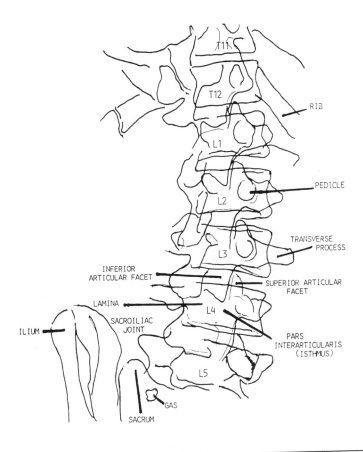

Posteroanterior Spot

L-5–S-1

Grid
40" SID (FFD)   80 kVp (optimum)

This film is best for the female patient. The patient's body can be used to protect the gonadal tissue. Obese patients may also be taken PA as this will help to flatten the abdomen.

- The patient is prone.
- The central ray is angled 20 to 30 degrees caudally. It enters the patient at the level of L-5.
- Collimate to a little less than film size. Measure on the angle of the central ray.
- Place the appropriate marker.

Anteroposterior Spot

L-5–S-1

Grid   80 kVp (optimum)
40" SID (FFD)   20 to 30 degree cephalic tube tilt

This film is best for males, due to gonad shield.

- Patient is supine.
- The central ray is angled 20 to 30 degrees cephalad, depending upon the sacral base angle. It enters approximately 2 inches above the superior margin of the symphysis pubis and exits at the level of the fifth lumbar vertebra.
- Be sure to place film accordingly, with the angle of the central ray.
- All other factors are the same as the PA spot view (above).

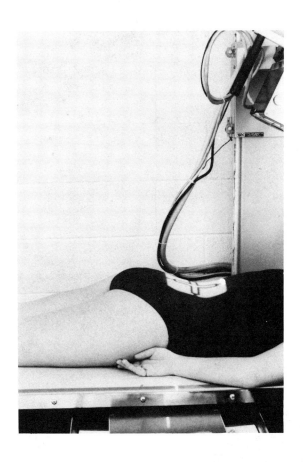

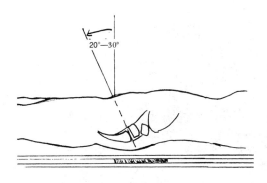

continued

Anteroposterior Spot: L-5–S-1

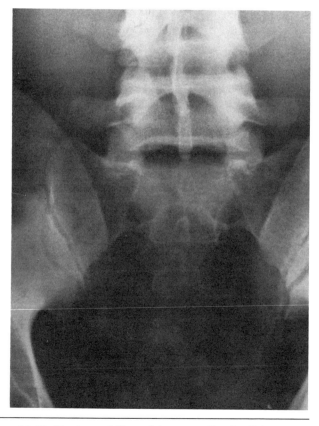

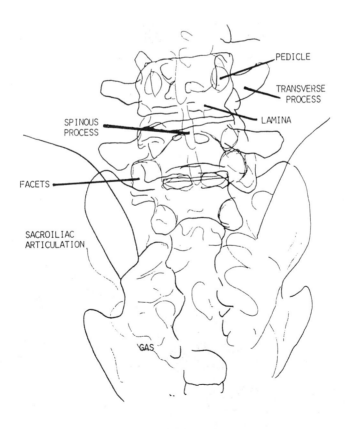

Anteroposterior Spot: L-5–S-1

Lateral Spot

Grid
40″ SID (FFD)

90 kVp (optimum)
8 × 10 film

This view is used to visualize the lumbosacral junction when not visualized on lateral view. It is especially helpful when there is a wide discrepancy between waist and hip measurements.

- The patient can be standing, seated, or side-lying. Remove as much rotation as possible.
- The central ray is 2 inches below the crest and approximately 4 inches anterior to the posterior body surface. (This may vary due to patient size.)
- Collimate to the posterior skin, unless there is considerable posterior adipose tissue, then move in accordingly and superiorly to a little less than film size.
- Measure through the central ray.
- Place the appropriate marker indicating the side closest to the film.

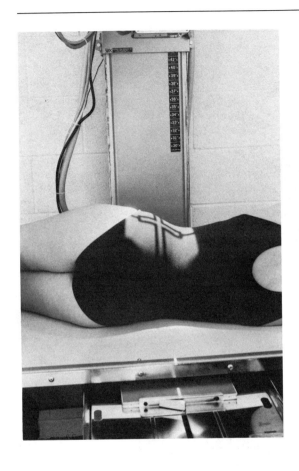

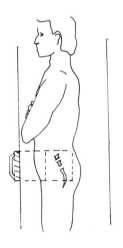

continued

Lateral Spot

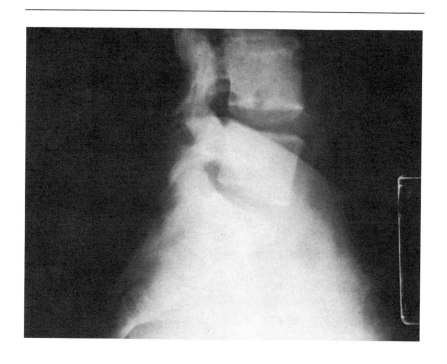
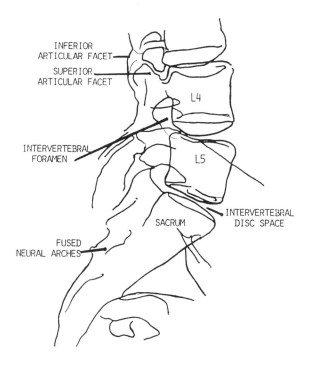

Full Spine

Anteroposterior Full Spine (For Scoliosis Evaluation)

Anteroposterior Full Spine (For Scoliosis Evaluation)

Grid
72 to 84" SID (FFD)
84 to 86 kVp (optimum)
14 × 36 cassette

- The patient is standing facing the tube with the feet directly under the hips. Sometimes it is helpful to place a mark on the floor so that the patient can align the heels with this to ensure proper placement.
- Have the patient open his or her mouth and position the head as if you were doing an APOM (the inferior margin of the incisors is parallel to the base of the occiput).
- Collimate to below the nose and to just below the symphysis pubis and laterally to a little less than film size. Place the cassette accordingly. This should place the central ray approximately at the xiphoid process.
- Measure sternum to spine and at the iliac crest level. Average these two measurements. Anyone measuring over 27 cm should be radiographed sectionally.
- Place the appropriate marker.
- It is felt by many that lateral views should be taken sectionally at all times.

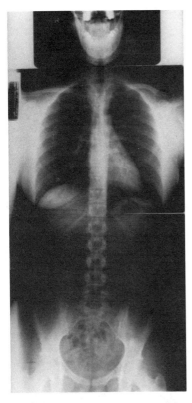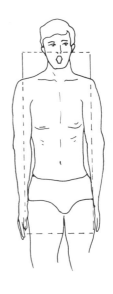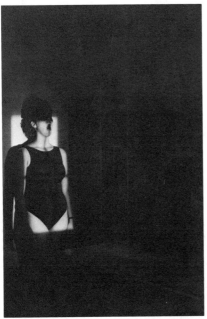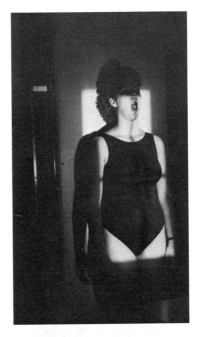

Anteroposterior Full Spine (For Scoliosis Evaluation)

Pelvis

Anteroposterior Pelvis

Anteroposterior Pelvis

Grid
40" SID (FFD)

80 kVp (optimum)
14 × 17 crosswise

- Patient is supine with feet rotated to midline and, if necessary, sandbagged. The film is placed so the top of the cassette is approximately 1 inch above the top of the iliac crest.
- Collimate to a little less than film size.
- Measure through the central ray.
- Place the appropriate marker, usually in the upper-outer corner.

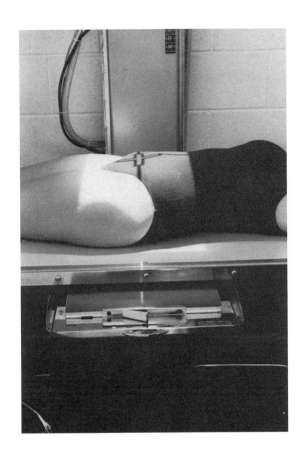

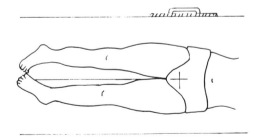

continued

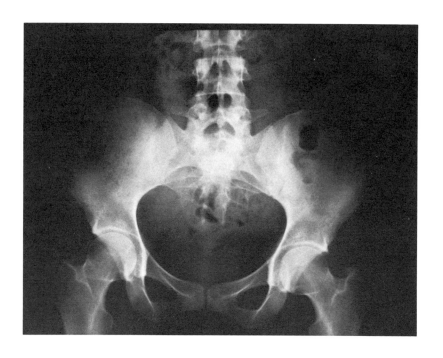

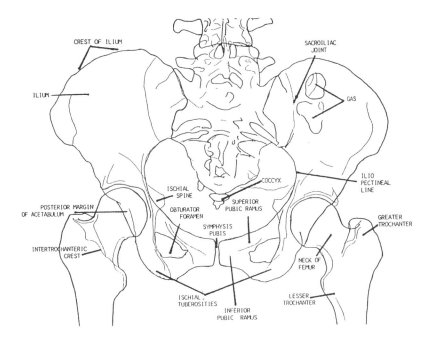

Hip

Anteroposterior Spot Hip
Frog Lateral

Anteroposterior Spot Hip

Grid
40" SID (FFD)

70 kVp (optimum)
10 × 12

- Patient is supine with foot rotated medially and, if necessary, sandbagged.
- The central ray is at the hip joint approximately 2 inches inferior and almost perpendicular to the midline of a line from the ASIS to the symphysis pubis.
- Collimate to a little less than film size.
- Measure through the central ray.
- Place the appropriate marker.

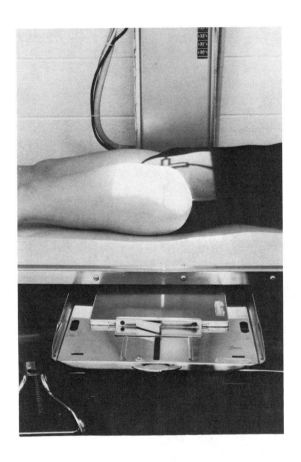

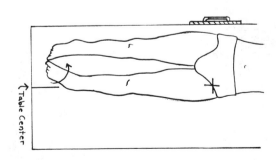

continued

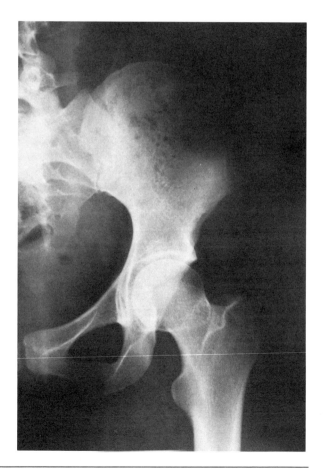

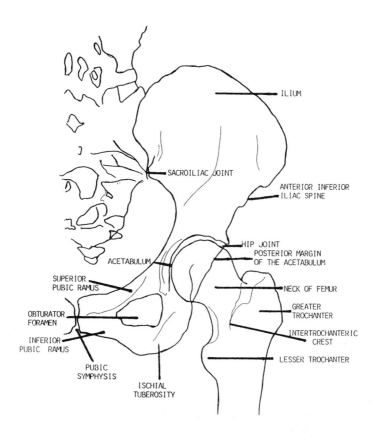

Frog Lateral

Grid
40″ SID (FFD)

66 kVp (optimum)
10 × 12 crosswise or an
11 × 14

- Patient is supine. Flex knee and place the foot under the popliteal fossa of the opposite leg, if possible. It may be necessary to rotate the opposite hip up to flatten the affected joint against the table.
- The central ray is at the crease formed at the joint.
- Collimate to a little less than film size.
- Measure through the central ray.
- Place the appropriate marker, usually in the upper-outer corner.

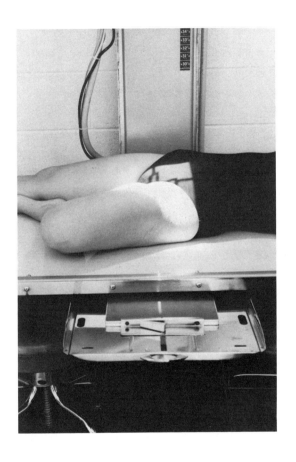

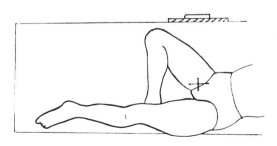

continued

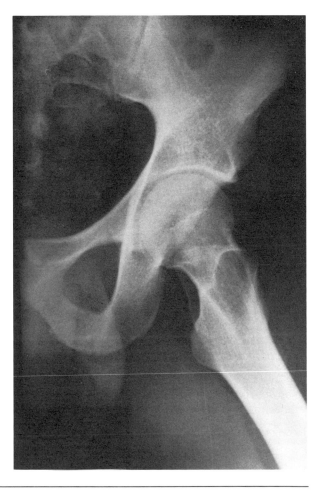

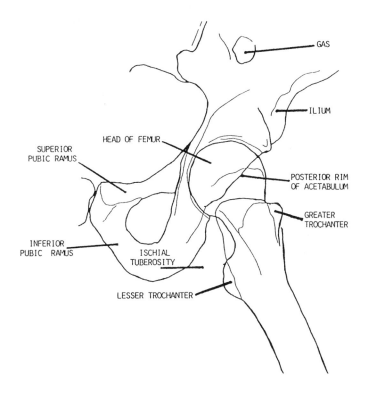

Frog Lateral

Sacrum

Anteroposterior Sacrum
Lateral Sacrum

Anteroposterior Sacrum

Grid
40″ SID (FFD)
15 degree cephalic tube tilt

70 kVp (optimum)
8 × 10 or 10 × 12

- Patient should evacuate and cleanse the bowel prior to the taking of the radiograph.
- The patient is supine.
- The central ray is angled 15 degrees cephalad and enters in the midline, half way between the symphysis pubis and the ASIS.
- Collimate to a little less than film size.
- Measure on the angle of the central ray.
- Place the appropriate marker.

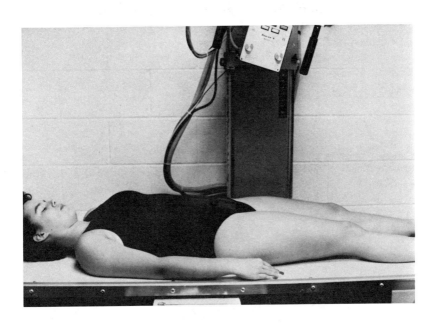
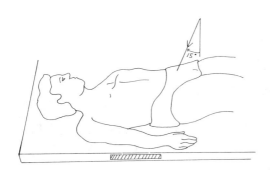

Lateral Sacrum

Grid
40″ SID (FFD)
90 kVp (optimum)
8 × 10

- The patient should evacuate and cleanse the bowel prior to the taking of the radiograph. The patient is standing or sidelying. Flex the hips and knees for support.
- Central ray is approximately 3 inches below the iliac crest.
- Collimate to the full length of the film and laterally to the posterior skin.
- Measure through the central ray.
- Place the appropriate marker.

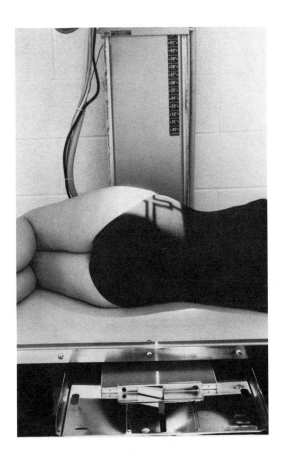

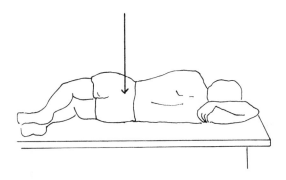

Lateral Sacrum

Coccyx

Anteroposterior Coccyx
Lateral Coccyx
Lateral Sacrum and Coccyx

Anteroposterior Coccyx

Grid
40" SID (FFD)
10 degree caudal tube tilt

70 kVp (optimum)
8 × 10

- Patient should evacuate and cleanse the bowel prior to the taking of the radiograph.
- The patient is supine.
- The central ray is angled 10 degrees caudally and placed in the midline 2½ inches above the symphysis pubis.
- Collimate a little less than film size.
- Measure on the angle of the central ray.
- Place the appropriate marker.

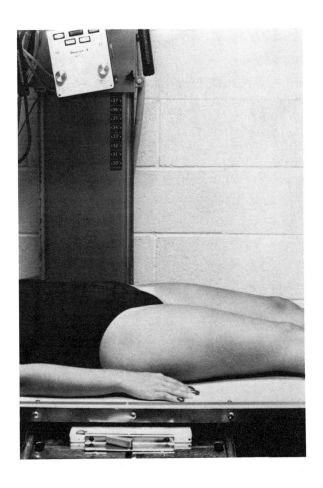

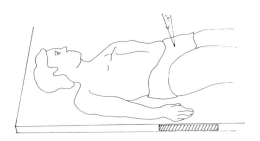

Anteroposterior Coccyx 85

Lateral Coccyx

Grid
40" SID (FFD)

80 kVp (optimum)
8 × 10

- The patient should evacuate and cleanse the bowel prior to the taking of the radiograph. The patient is standing or side-lying. Flex the hips and knees for support.
- Central ray is approximately 4 to 5 inches below the iliac crest.
- Collimate to the full length of the film and laterally to the posterior skin.
- Measure through the central ray.
- Place the appropriate marker.

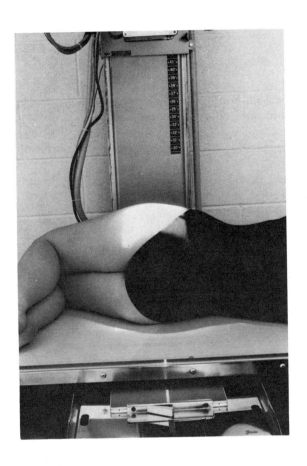
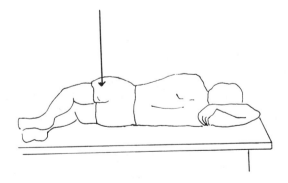

Lateral Coccyx

Lateral Sacrum and Coccyx

Grid 86 kVp (optimum)
40" SID (FFD) 10 × 12

- The patient should evacuate and cleanse the bowel prior to the taking of the radiograph. The patient is standing or side-lying. Flex the hips and knees for support of side-lying.
- The central ray is approximately 3 to 4 inches below the iliac crest, and approximately 2 inches anterior to the posterior skin.
- Collimate to the full length of the film and laterally to the posterior skin.
- Measure through the central ray.
- Place the appropriate marker.

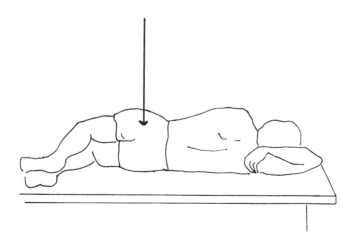

Knee

Anteroposterior Knee
Posteroanterior Knee
Lateral Knee
Tunnel View
Tangential (Sunrise)

Either the AP or PA view may be taken. Up to 17 cm either grid or non-grid is acceptable; over 17 cm must be grid.

Anteroposterior Knee

Non-Grid
Grid
40″ SID (FFD)
5 degree cephalic tube tilt

50 kVp (optimum)
70 kVp (optimum)
8 × 10 unless patient is extremely large, if this is the case then use a 10 × 12

- Patient is supine. The extremity is fully extended, with the foot perpendicular to the table.
- The central ray is angled 5 degrees cephalad and enters at the inferior margin of the patella.
- Collimate to a little less than film size.
- Measure on the angle of the central ray.
- Place the appropriate marker.

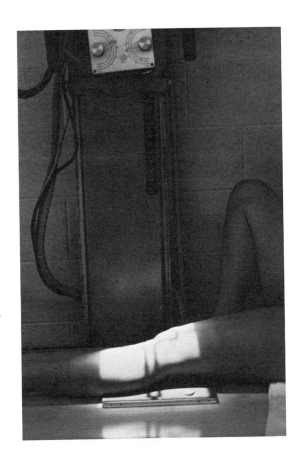

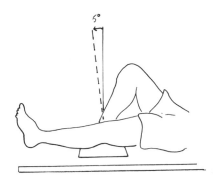

Anteroposterior Knee

Posteroanterior Knee

Non-Grid
Grid
40" SID (FFD)

50 kVp (optimum)
70 kVp (optimum)
8 × 10 unless patient is extremely large, if this is the case then use a 10 × 12

- Patient is prone. The extremity is fully extended and the ankle extends over the end of the surface of the table.
- The central ray is directed to exit at the center of the patella.
- Collimate to a little less than film size.
- Measure through the central ray.
- Place the appropriate marker.

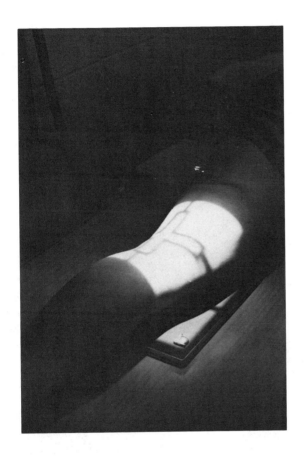

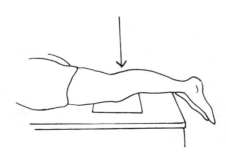

continued

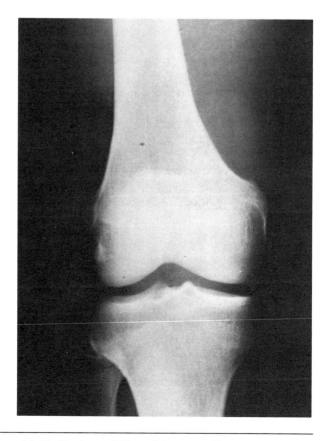

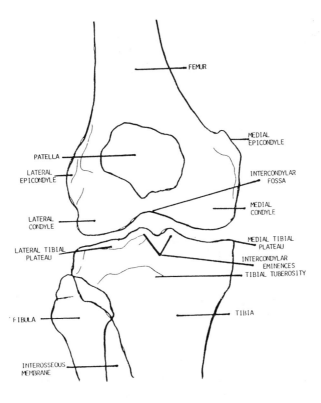

Lateral Knee

Non-Grid
Grid
40" SID (FFD)
10 to 12 degree cephalic tube tilt

50 kVp (optimum)
70 kVp (optimum)
8 × 10 unless patient is extremely large, if this is the case then use a 10 × 12

- The patient is side-lying with the affected limb down (lateral surface of affected limb on cassette). The top leg is brought forward and may be cushioned with a pillow. This allows you to flatten the affected knee to the cassette and stabilize the patient.
- The long axis of the film is parallel to the long axis of the thigh (femur).
- The knee is flexed about 45 degrees extending off the corner of the cassette.
- The central ray is angled approximately 12 degrees cephalad through the joint space.
- Collimate to a little less than film size.
- Measure on the angle through the central ray.
- Be sure to place the cassette in line with the central ray.

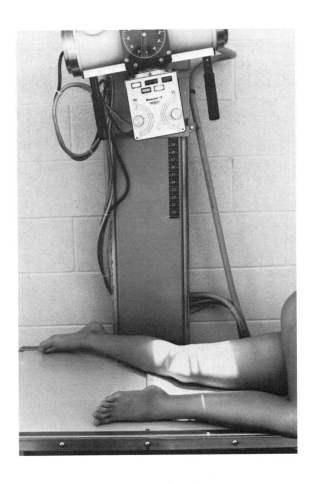

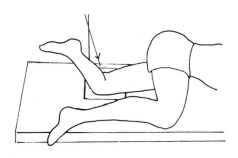

continued

Lateral Knee

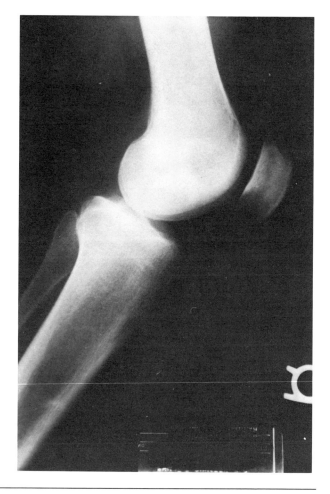

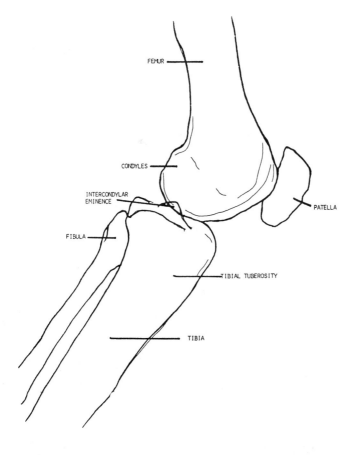

Tunnel View

Non-Grid
Grid
40" SID (FFD)
45 degree caudal tube tilt

50 kVp (optimum)
70 kVp (optimum)
8 × 10 unless patient is extremely large, if this is the case then use a 10 × 12

- The patient is prone. The knee is flexed 45 degrees.
- The central ray is angled 45 degrees caudally, emerging through the bottom of the patella. Be sure to compensate for the tube tilt by lowering the tube 1 inch for each 5 degrees of tilt (this avoids magnification).
- Collimate to a little less than film size. Increase kVp 4 to 6 from AP or PA.
- Place the appropriate marker.
- Be sure to place the cassette in line with the tube tilt (approximately 1 inch to 1½ inches of femur is on the cassette).

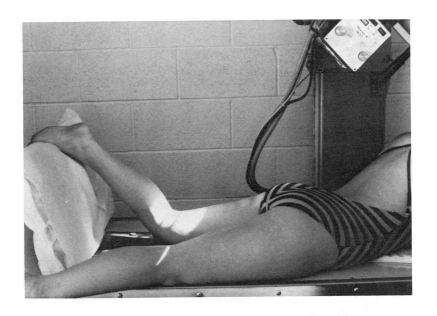

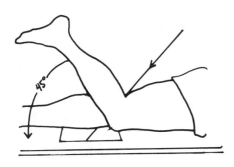

continued

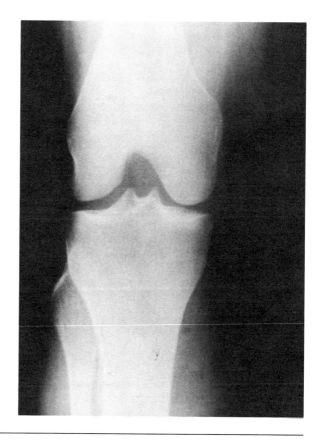

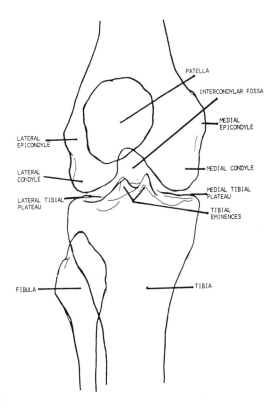

Tunnel View

Tangential (Sunrise)

Non-Grid
Grid
40" SID (FFD)

50 kVp (optimum)
70 kVp (optimum)
8 × 10 unless patient is extremely large, if this is the case then use a 10 × 12

- The patient is prone. The knee is in extreme flexion.
- The central ray is 2 inches superior to the most anterior surface of the patella.
- Collimate to include the patella (smaller than film size).
- Place the appropriate marker.
- If the patient cannot fully flex the leg, a cephalad tube tilt will need to be employed.

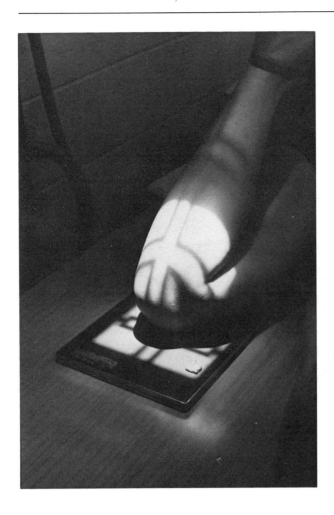

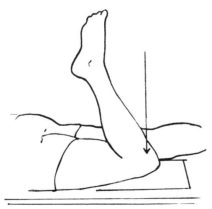

continued

Tangential (Sunrise) 105

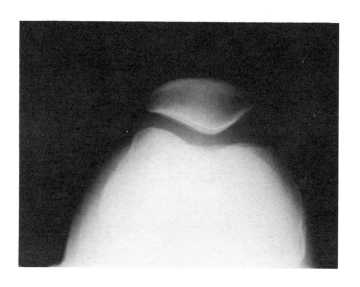

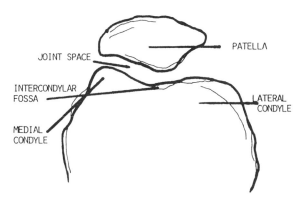

Ankle

Anteroposterior Ankle
Medial Oblique Ankle (Mortise View)
Lateral Ankle

Anteroposterior Ankle

Non-Grid
40″ SID (FFD)

50 kVp (optimum)
½ of 8 × 10 or 10 × 12

- The patient is lying or sitting. Leg is fully extended and foot is 90 degrees to leg.
- The central ray is at the level of the malleoli in the midline, through the joint space.
- Collimate to the size of the area of film being utilized.
- Measure through the central ray.
- Place the appropriate marker. Only one view on the cassette needs to be marked.

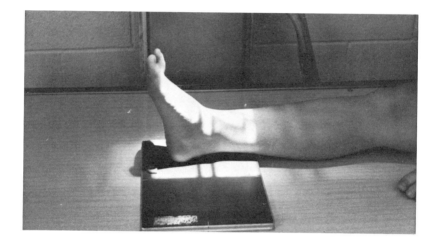

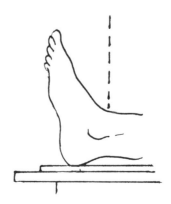

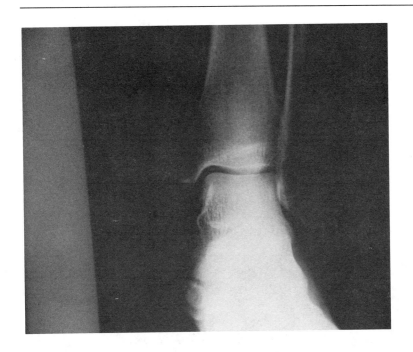

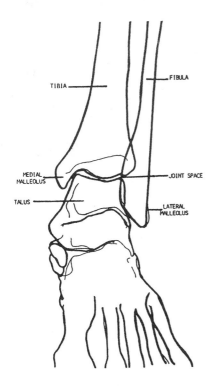

Anteroposterior Ankle

Medial Oblique Ankle (Mortise View)

Non-Grid
40" SID (FFD)

50 kVp (optimum)
½ of 8 × 10 or 10 × 12

- The patient is lying or sitting. The leg is fully extended. The foot is perpendicular to the leg. The foot is rotated until a line drawn through the malleoli is parallel to the cassette.
- The central ray is at the level of the malleoli.
- Collimate to the size of the area of the film being utilized.
- Use the same factors as the AP.

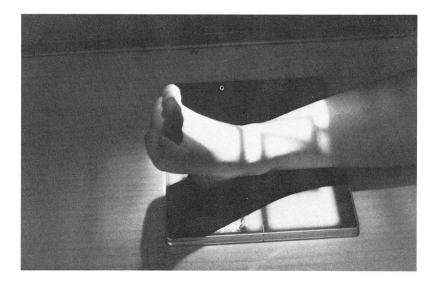

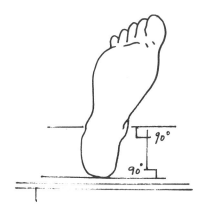

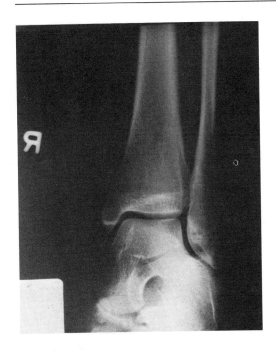

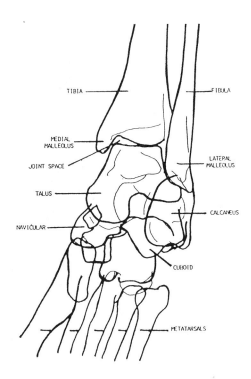

Medial Oblique Ankle (Mortise View)

Lateral Ankle

Non-Grid
40" SID (FFD)

50 kVp (optimum)
8 × 10 film

- The patient is side-lying with the lateral surface of the affected limb down, the opposite leg is brought forward to help stabilize (similar to the position of a lateral knee projection). The foot is at 90 degrees to the leg.
- The central ray is at the level of the malleolus.
- Collimate to include the needed structures.
- Measure through the central ray.
- Place the appropriate marker.

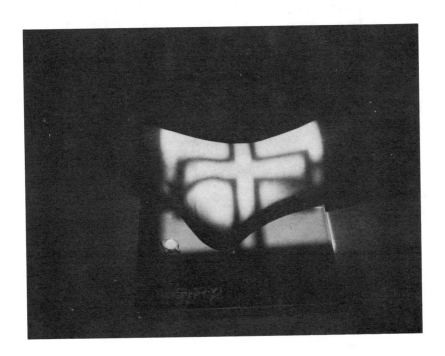

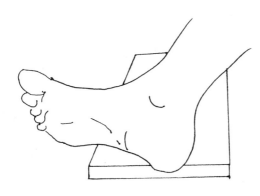

continued

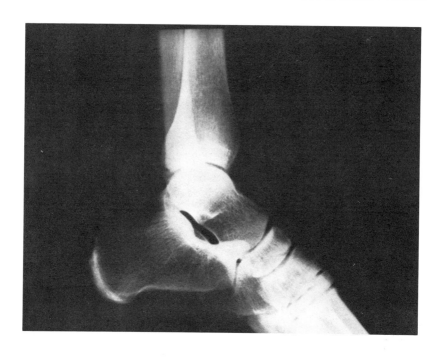

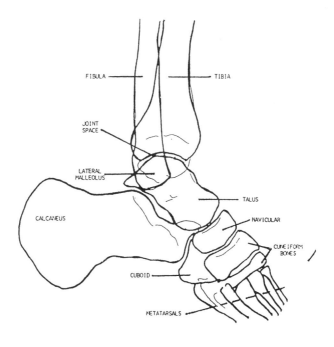

Foot

Dorsoplantar Foot (AP)
Medial Oblique Foot
Lateral Foot

Dorsoplantar Foot (AP)

Non-Grid 50 kVp (optimum)
40" SID (FFD)
5 degree cephalic tube tilt

Film size is dependent upon patient foot size. The object of a foot series is to visualize all of the structures of the foot.

- The foot is placed with the plantar surface flat on the cassette.
- The central ray is angled 5 degrees and enters in the center of the foot at the more proximal aspect of the metatarsals. Allow for visualization of all of the toes.
- Collimate to the size of the area of the film being utilized.
- Measure on the angle of the central ray.
- Place the appropriate marker.

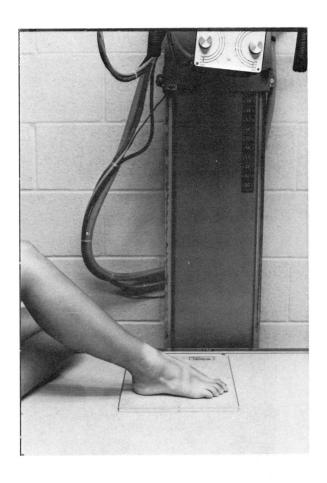

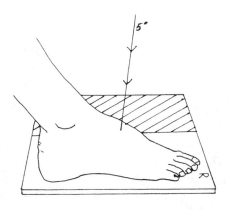

continued

Dorsoplantar Foot (AP) 117

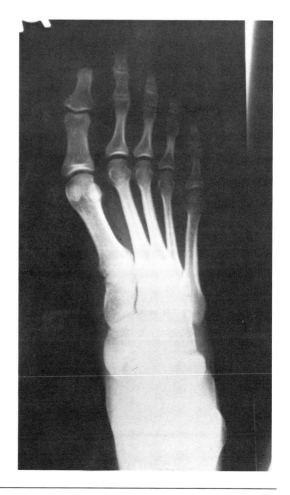

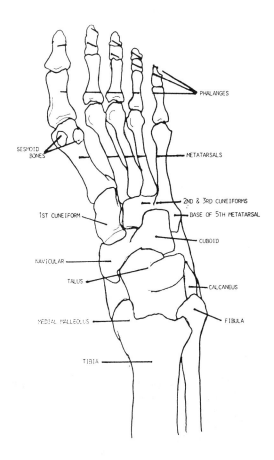

Dorsoplantar Foot (AP)

Medial Oblique Foot

Non-Grid 50 kVp (optimum)
40″ SID (FFD)

- The patient must rotate the entire leg (calf) and foot 45 degrees medially.
- Central ray is in the middle of the foot at the more proximal aspect of the metatarsals. All of the toes must be included.
- Collimate to the size of the area of film being utilized.
- Measure through the central ray.

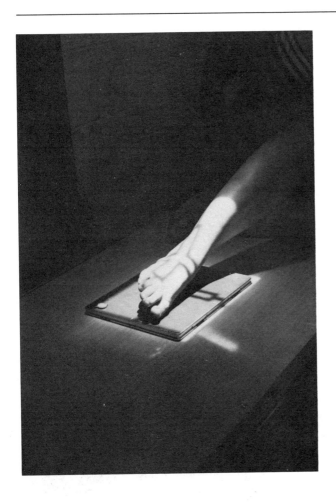

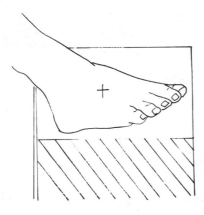

continued

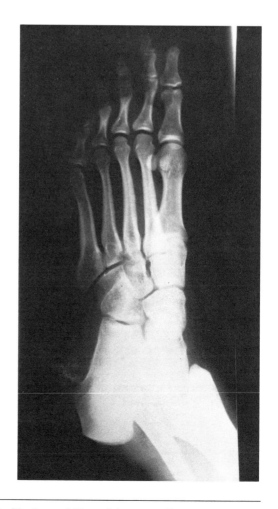

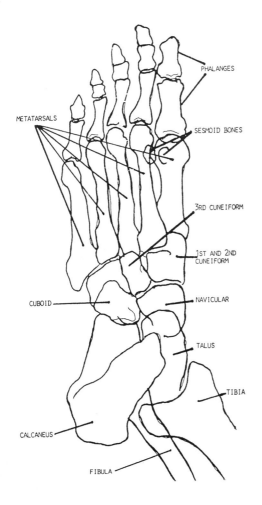

Medial Oblique Foot

Lateral Foot

Non-Grid
40" SID (FFD)

50 kVp (optimum)
½ of 10 × 12 or appropriate film size

- The foot is placed at 90 degrees to the leg, with the lateral surface of the affected limb against the cassette.
- Central ray is through the middle of the foot.
- Collimate to include all of the foot. Both the toes and the calcaneus must be visualized in their entirety.
- Measure through the central ray.
- Place the appropriate marker.

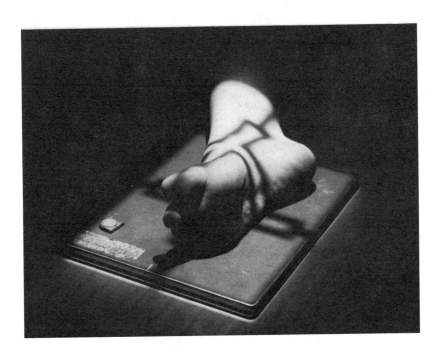

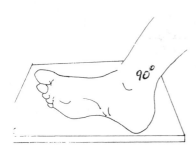

continued

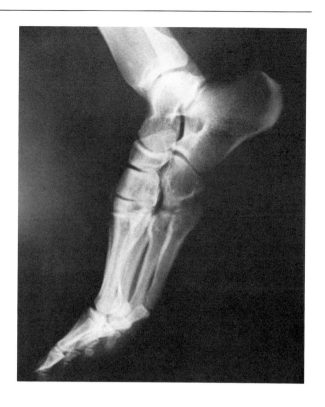

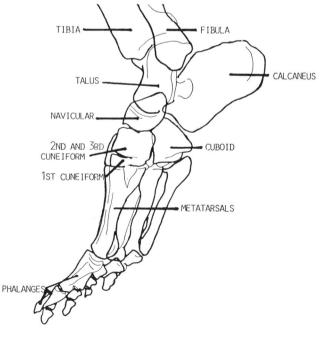

Toes

Dorsoplantar Toes (AP)
Oblique Toes

Dorsoplantar Toes (AP)

Non-Grid
40" SID (FFD)

44 to 46 kVp (optimum)
½ of 8 × 10 or 10 × 12, depending on foot size and width

- The foot is placed flat on the cassette.
- The central ray is through the third digit.
- Collimate to include the phalanges and metatarsals.
- Measure through the central ray.
- Place the appropriate marker.

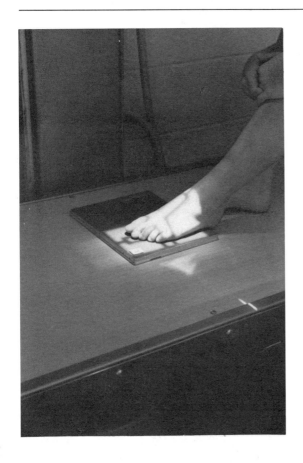

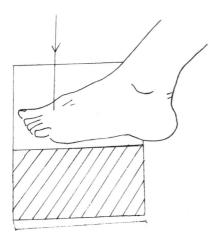

Dorsoplantar Toes (AP) 129

Oblique Toes

Non-Grid 44 to 46 kVp (optimum)
40″ SID (FFD) ½ of 8 × 10 or 10 × 12

- Place the foot in the dorsoplantar position and then rotate the foot and leg 45 degrees medially.
- The central ray is through the third digit.
- Collimate to include the phalanges and metatarsals.
- Measure through the central ray.
- Place the appropriate marker; only one view of this series needs to be marked.

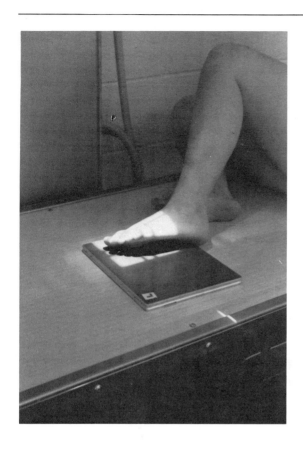

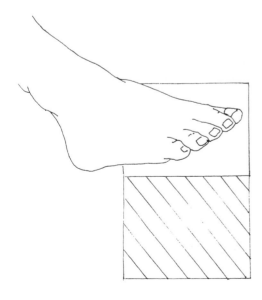

Oblique Toes 131

Calcaneus

Plantodorsal Calcaneus
  Tangential
Lateral Calcaneus

Plantodorsal Calcaneus

Tangential

Non-Grid 50 kVp (optimum)
40″ SID (FFD) ½ of 8 × 10
35 to 40 degree caudal tube tilt

- The foot is flexed 90 degrees to the leg. It may be necessary for the patient to use a cord to hold the foot in this position.
- The central ray is angled 35 to 40 degrees caudad and is through the calcaneus, approximately 2 inches above its base, however, this will vary with the foot size. Be sure to compensate for the tube tilt by lowering the tube 1 inch for each 5 degrees of tilt, to avoid magnification. Collimate to the size of the area of the film being utilized. Measure on the angle of the central ray and place the film accordingly.
- Place the appropriate marker. This is often the view that has the marker and film blocker.

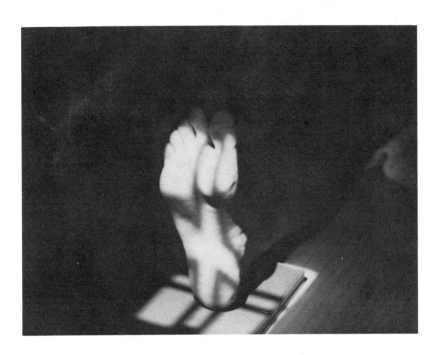

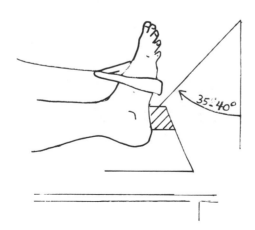

Plantodorsal Calcaneus: Tangential

Lateral Calcaneus

Non-Grid
40" SID (FFD)

50 kVp (optimum)
½ of 8 × 10

- The affected leg is down with the lateral surface of the calcaneus against the cassette. The foot is at 90 degrees to the leg.
- The central ray is in the center of the calcaneus.
- Collimate to the size of the area being utilized.
- Measure through the central ray.

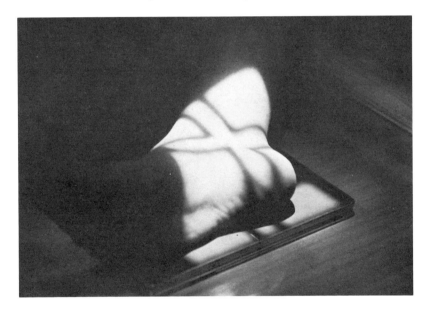

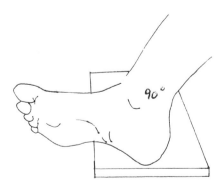

Shoulder

External Rotation (AP)
Internal Rotation
Stress View (AP)

External Rotation (AP)

Grid   70 kVp (optimum)
40" SID (FFD)   10 × 12 crosswise

- The patient is supine or upright. Turn the patient's head away from the affected shoulder.
- Externally rotate the patient's arm, making sure you truly rotate the arm and that the patient does not just pronate or supinate the hand.
- The central ray is at the coracoid process.
- Collimate to a little less than film size.
- Measure through the central ray.
- Place the appropriate marker.

Internal Rotation

This view is positioned the same as the External Rotation, except the arm is now internally rotated.

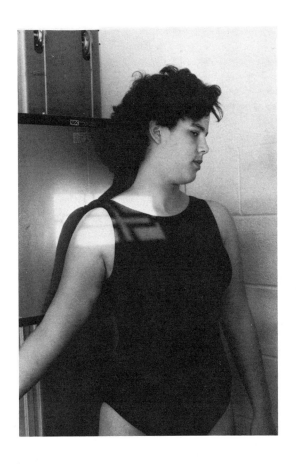

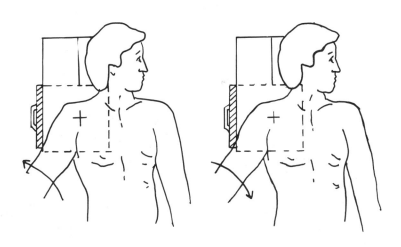

continued

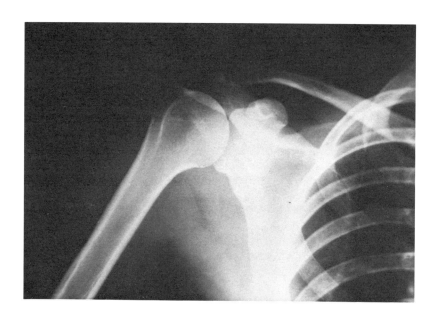

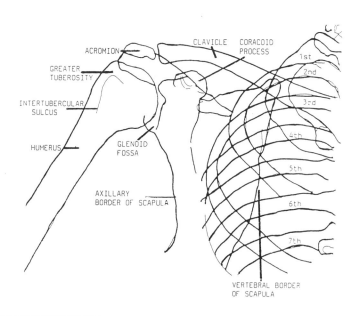

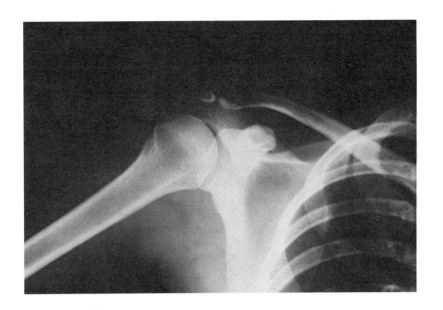

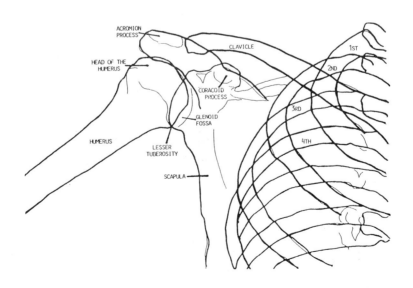

Stress View (AP)

Wall grid
40" SID (FFD)
Weight: approximately 15 lb for females; 25 lb for males

70 kVp (optimum)
8 × 10

- Patient is facing the X-ray tube with the head turned. He or she moves laterally and stands so the coracoid process is at the center of the grid. The patient is holding the appropriate weight.
- The central ray is at the coracoid process.
- Collimate to a little less than film size.
- Measure through the central ray.
- Place the appropriate marker.

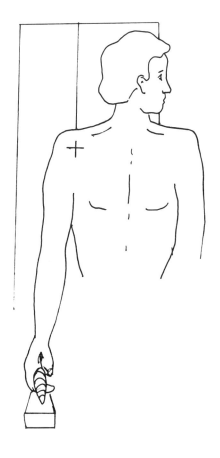

Elbow

Anteroposterior Elbow
Medial Oblique Elbow
Lateral Elbow
Tangential Elbow (Jones' View)

Anteroposterior Elbow

Non-Grid
40" SID (FFD)
50 kVp (optimum)
¼ of 10 × 12

- The patient is seated comfortably at the X-ray table. The arm and forearm are in full extension, lying flat against the cassette. The palm is up (supinate the hand).
- The central ray is at the antecubital fossa.
- Collimate to the size of the area of the film being utilized.
- Measure through the central ray.
- Place an appropriate marker on the film, usually on the quarter used for the tangential (Jones') view, since there is more space. The film blocker is also often in this area.

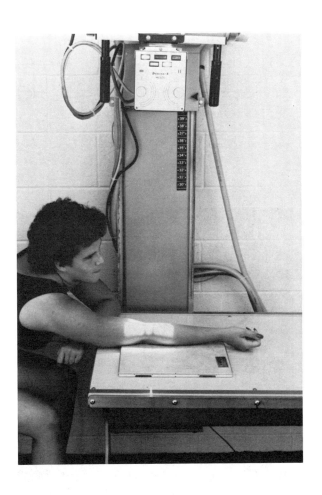

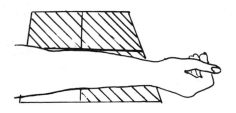

continued

Anteroposterior Elbow

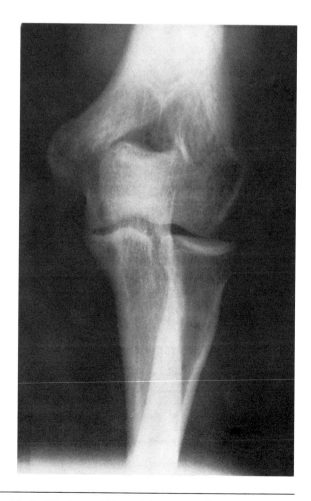

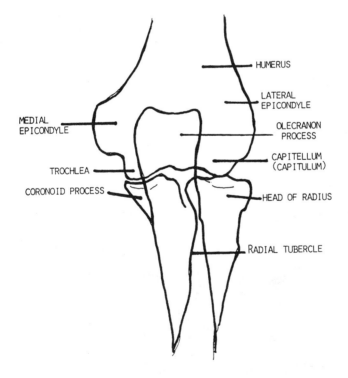

Medial Oblique Elbow

Non-Grid 50 kVp (optimum)
40″ SID (FFD) ¼ of 10 × 12

- The patient is seated at the X-ray table. The arm is in full extension. The arm and forearm lay flat against the cassette. The palm is down (pronate the hand).
- The central ray is at the antecubital fossa.
- Collimate to the size of the area of the film being utilized.
- Measure through the central ray.

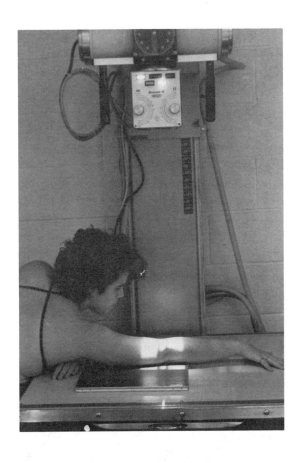

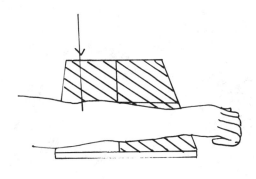

continued

Medial Oblique Elbow 149

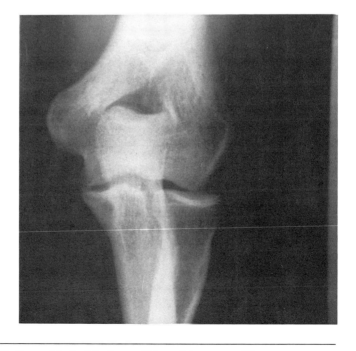

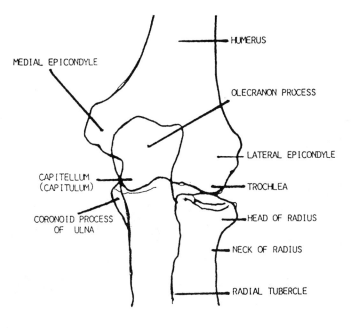

Lateral Elbow

Non-Grid
40″ SID (FFD)

50 kVp (optimum)
¼ of 10 × 12

- The patient is seated at the X-ray table. The elbow is flexed 90 degrees and the hand and wrist are placed in the true lateral position. The humerus is parallel with the table (shoulder down). The thumb is up.
- The central ray is at the middle of the joint space.
- Collimate to the size of the area of the film being utilized.
- Measure through the central ray.

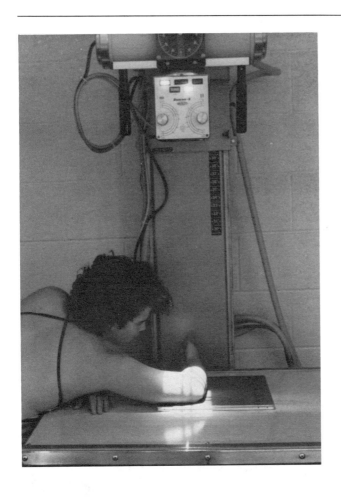

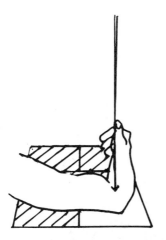

continued

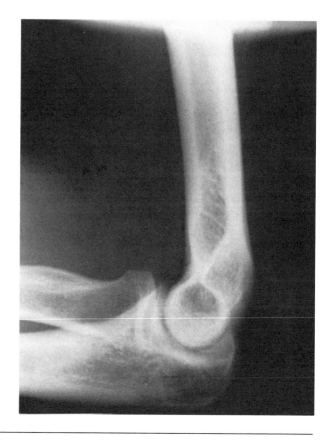

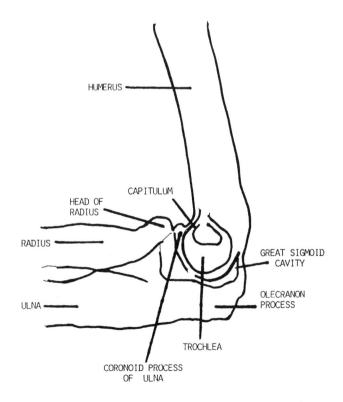

Tangential Elbow (Jones' View)

Non-Grid 50 kVp (optimum)
40″ SID (FFD) ¼ of 10 × 12

- The patient is seated at the X-ray table. The elbow is flexed with the hand placed on the patient's shoulder or to the patient's tolerance.
- The central ray is placed 2 inches above the end of the olecranon process. If the patient cannot fully flex the elbow, a cephalad tube tilt may be needed. Collimate to the size of the area of the film being utilized.
- Measure through the central ray.
- The marker and film blocker are often in this quadrant.

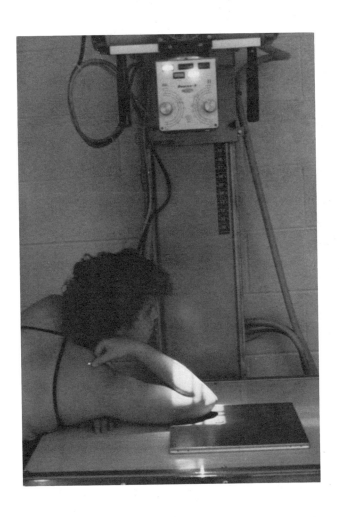

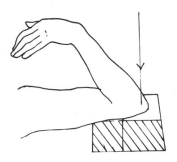

continued

Tangential Elbow

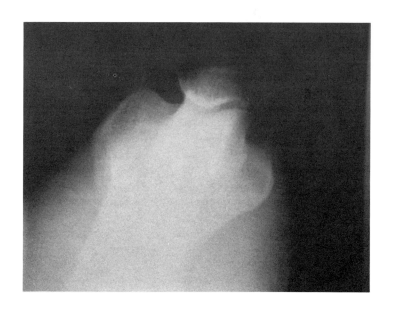

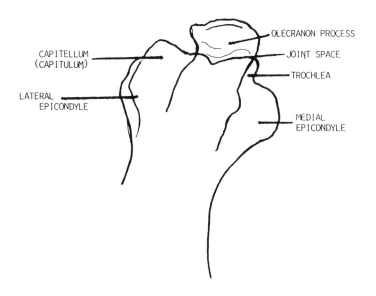

Forearm

Anteroposterior Forearm
Lateral Forearm

The joint nearest the injury *must always* be included, however, it is best if both joints can be included.

Anteroposterior Forearm

Non-Grid
40" SID (FFD)

50 kVp (optimum)
Cassette size varies with the size of the extremity

- The patient is seated and the arm is supinated. The wrist and elbow joints are extended.
- The central ray is at the middle of the forearm.
- Collimate to include all bony and soft tissue structures.
- Measure through the central ray.

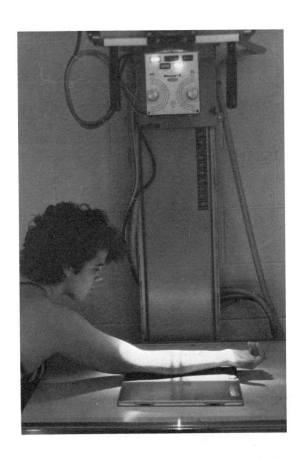
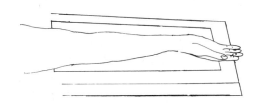

Anteroposterior Forearm

Lateral Forearm

Non-Grid
40" SID (FFD)

50 kVp (optimum)
Cassette size will vary with the size of the extremity

- The patient's arm is placed in the same manner as in a lateral elbow view with the wrist in a true lateral position.
- The central ray is at the middle of the forearm.
- Collimate to include all bony and soft tissue structures.
- Measure through the central ray.
- Place the appropriate marker.

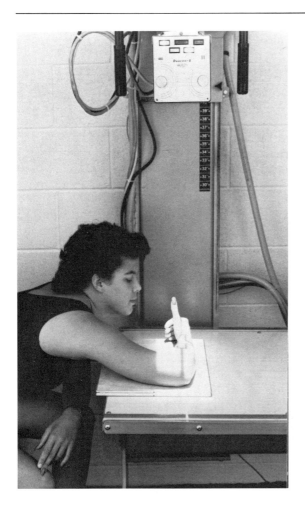

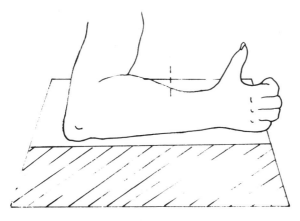

Lateral Forearm

Wrist

Posteroanterior Wrist
Dorsopalmar
Oblique Wrist
Posteroanterior
Lateral Wrist
Supplemental
Radial and Ulnar Deviation Views
Carpal Tunnel View

Posteroanterior

Dorsopalmar

Non-Grid   50 kVp (optimum)
40" SID (FFD)   ⅓ of 10 × 12

- Place the wrist in the prone position, palm down. The patient's hand is brought up into a loose fist to flatten the wrist against the film.
- The central ray is at the middle of the wrist (mid-portion of the carpal bones).
- Collimate to the size of the area of film being utilized. Measure through the central ray.
- Place the appropriate marker. The marker needs to be placed only on one view of the series. This is usually the lateral view because there is more space.

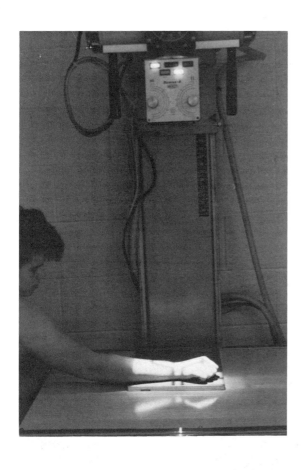

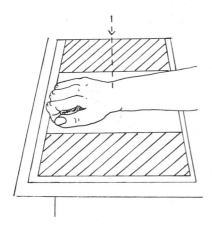

continued

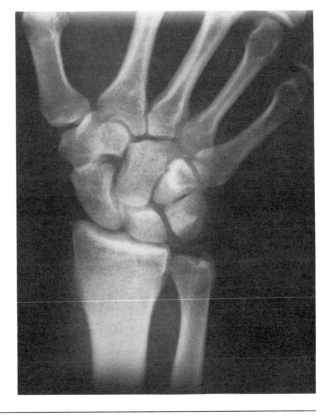

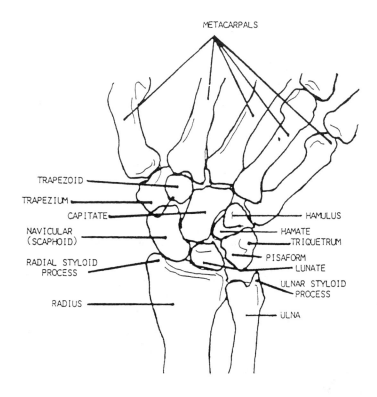

Oblique Wrist

Posteroanterior

Non-Grid 50 kVp (optimum)
40″ SID (FFD) ⅓ of 10 × 12

- Place the patient's hand in the prone position (dorsopalmar). The hand and forearm are in the same plane. Rotate the wrist laterally 45 degrees. You may use a wedge to rest the wrist upon or use the thumb for support. The hand, as in the posteroanterior view, is in a loose fist.
- The central ray is at the middle of the wrist.
- Collimate to the size of the area of film being utilized.
- Measure through the central ray.

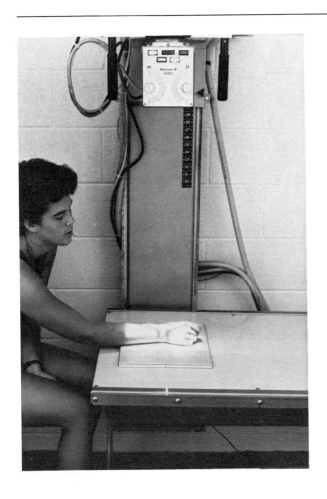

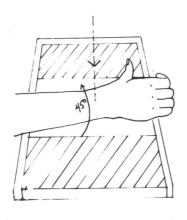

continued

Oblique Wrist: Posteroanterior

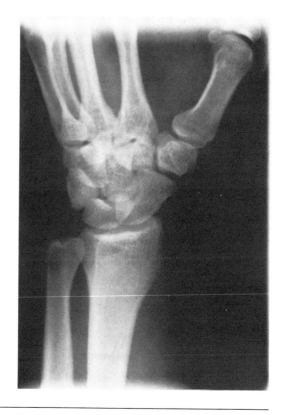

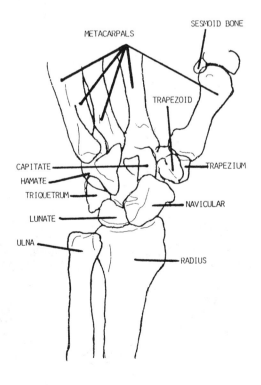

Oblique Wrist: Posteroanterior

Lateral Wrist

Non-Grid
40″ SID (FFD)

50 kVp (optimum)
⅓ of 10 × 12

- Place the patient's wrist so that the forearm and hand are in the same plane, perpendicular to the cassette. Place the thumb up.
- The central ray is at the middle of the wrist.
- Collimate to the size of the area of film being utilized.
- Measure through the central ray.

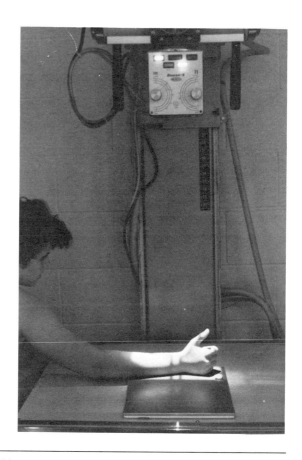

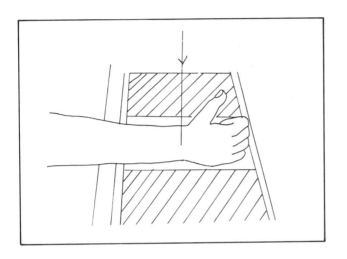

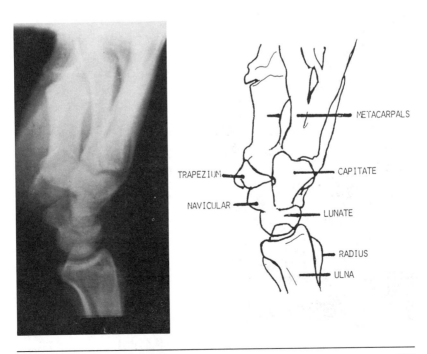

Lateral Wrist

Supplemental

Radial and Ulnar Deviation Views

Non-Grid   50 kVp (optimum)
40″ SID (FFD)   ½ of 8 × 10

- The patient's wrist is in the prone position (palm down). Ulnar flex or radially flex the wrist as far as possible.
- The central ray is at the middle of the wrist.
- Collimate to the size of the area of film being utilized.
- Measure through the central ray.
- Place the appropriate marker.

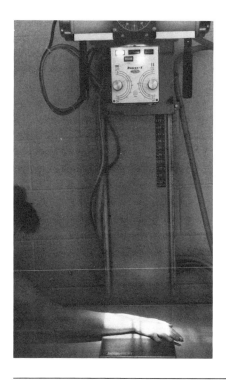
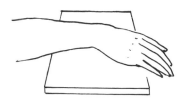

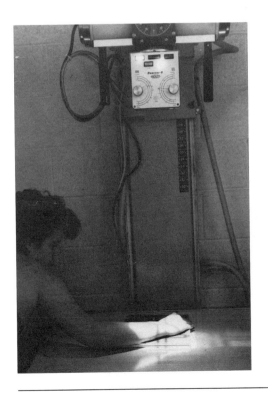 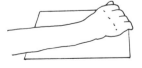

Carpal Tunnel View

Non-Grid
40" SID (FFD)
45 degree caudal tube tilt

50 kVp (optimum)
8 × 10

- The patient is seated. The hand is at 90 degrees (or as close to this as possible) to the wrist and the anterior aspect of the wrist is flat on the cassette. The central ray enters on the palmar side at a caudal angle of 45 degrees through the center of the carpal tunnel, distal to proximal.
- Collimate to include the area being filmed.
- Measure on the angle of the central ray.
- Place the appropriate marker.
- Occasionally it is easier to achieve maximum dorsiflexion of the hand if the palm lies on the cassette and the arm is brought forward (over the hand). The patient is seated or standing.
- The central ray enters the carpal tunnel proximal to distal at a 45 degree caudal angle.

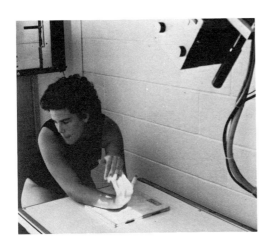
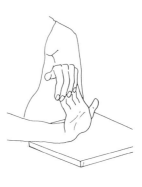

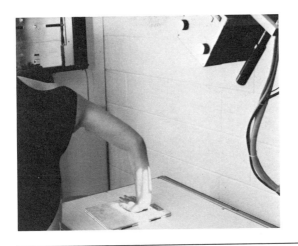
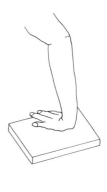

Hand

Dorsopalmar Hand (PA)
Oblique Hand
Lateral Hand

Dorsopalmar Hand (PA)

Non-Grid
40" SID (FFD)

50 kVp (optimum)
Film size determined by patient hand size

Be sure you allow for visualization of all the distal phalanges.

- Patient is seated comfortably at the X-ray table. The hand is flat on the cassette. Fingers are spread apart.
- Central ray is in the middle of the hand (not necessarily in the middle of the metacarpals).
- Collimate to include the entire hand.
- Measure through the central ray.
- Place the appropriate marker. The patient ID should be placed in the area near the wrist.

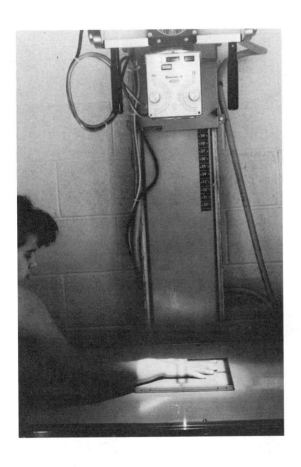

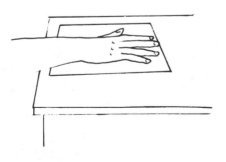

continued

Dorsopalmar Hand (PA)

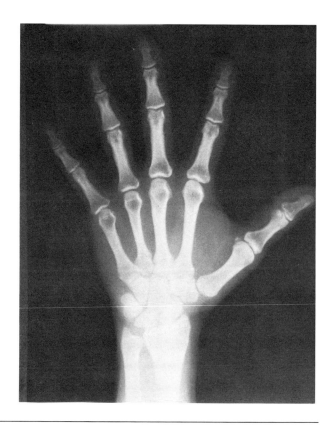

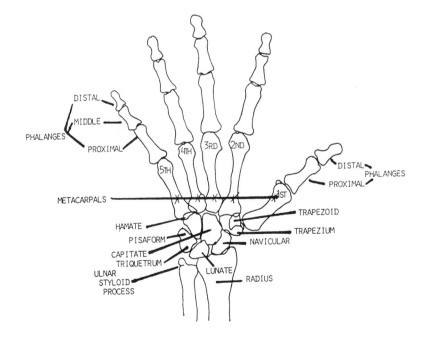

Oblique Hand

Non-Grid
40" SID (FFD)

50 kVp (optimum)
Film size determined by patient hand size

- Place the hand with the pisiform (inferolateral aspect of hand) on the cassette and spread the fingers.
- The central ray is in the middle of the hand.
- Collimate to include the entire hand. Use PA measurement.
- Place the appropriate marker.

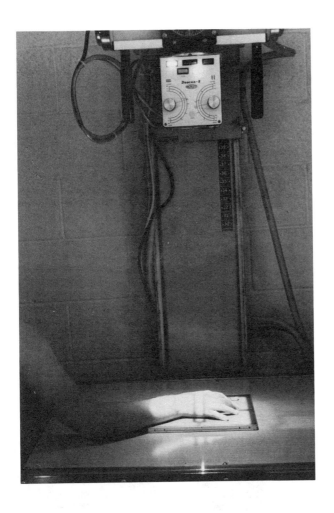

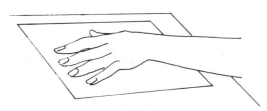

continued

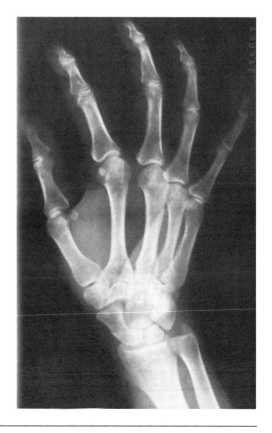

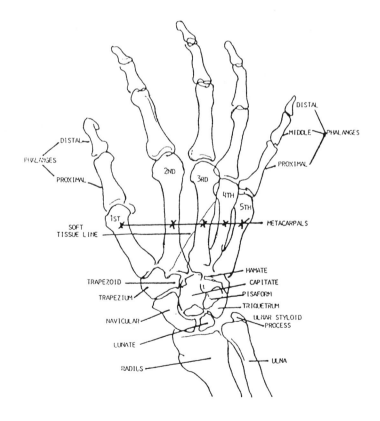

Oblique Hand

Lateral Hand

Non-Grid
40" SID (FFD)

50 kVp (optimum)
8 × 10 or larger depending on hand size

- Be sure all digits are totally visualized.
- Place hand in the lateral position so hand and forearm are in the same plane. Place the fingers so no finger superimposes another.
- Central ray is through the middle of the hand, approximately the head of the second metacarpal.
- Collimate to include all of the fingers.
- Place the appropriate marker.

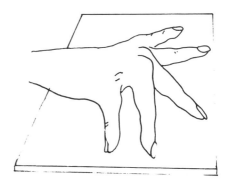

Fingers

Finger Series

Finger Series

Non-Grid
40″ SID (FFD)

50 kVp for hand decrease kVp 2 to 4 or one time station for the digits

First do a (PA) hand. Several projections of one digit can be done on an 8 × 10. Various methods of positioning the individual digits are illustrated. You should try to do at least a posteroanterior, lateral, and one oblique view. It is more complete if both the medial and lateral oblique views are obtained.

- Collimate to include the digit.
- Place an appropriate marker on the film.

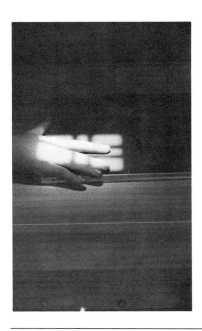
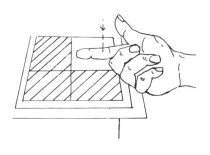

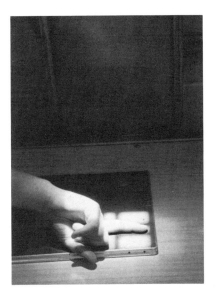
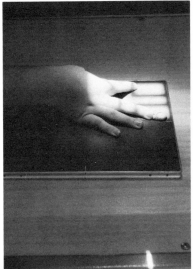
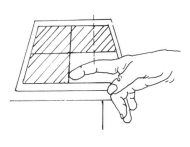
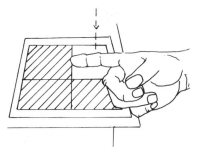

Finger Series

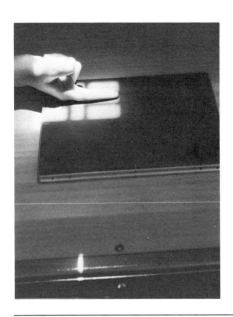
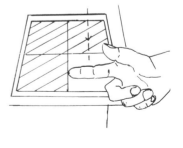

Skull

Caldwell's Projection
  Posteroanterior Caldwell
Anteroposterior Towne's
  Occipital
Lateral Skull
Axial View of Skull
  Base-Vertex, Submento-Vertex

Be sure to check that there is no rotation or tilt to the patient's head in all skull views. Be sure that the patient removes all possible artifacts, including contacts, hairpins, wigs, etc.

Caldwell's Projection

Posteroanterior Caldwell

Grid
40" SID (FFD)
15 degree caudal tube tilt

84 to 90 kVp (optimum)
10 × 12

- Patient is prone. Adjust patient's head so the canthomeatal line is perpendicular to the table. Having the patient tuck their chin may be helpful.
- Central ray is angled 15 degrees caudally and exits at the glabella, the bony prominence on the frontal bone joining the supraorbital ridges.
- Collimate to a little less than film size.
- Measure through the angle of the central ray.
- Place the appropriate marker.
- If using a Supertech, this view is figured on the second line under the skull.
- Add 1½ to the machine CF for skull series (e.g., minus 1½ for skull, plus 1 for the machine = TCF − ½).

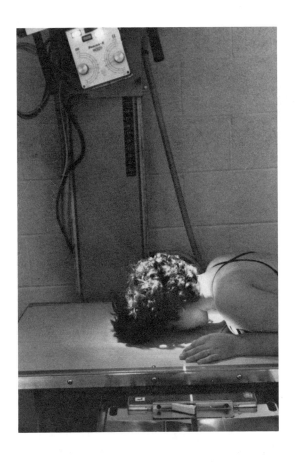

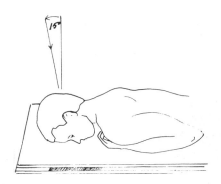

continued

Caldwell's Projection: Posteroanterior Caldwell   197

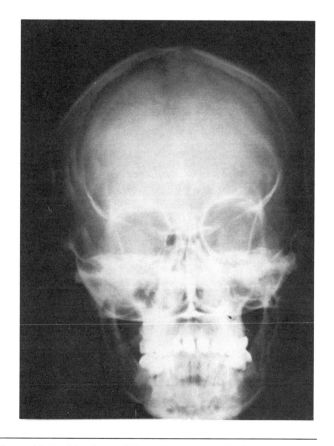

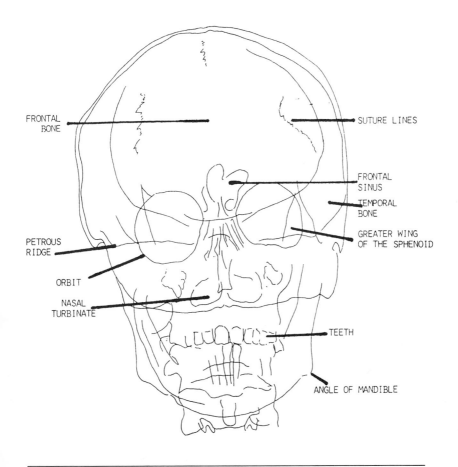

Anteroposterior Towne's

Occipital

Grid 84 to 90 kVp
40" SID (FFD) 10 × 12
35 degree caudal tube tilt

- Patient is supine. Head is placed so the canthomeatal line is perpendicular to the table. Bring the patient's chin down.
- Central ray is angled 35 degrees caudally, enters in the midline approximately 3 inches above the superior boundary of the orbits, and exits at the level of the EOP.
- Collimate a little less than film size.
- Measure on the angle of the central ray, place the cassette accordingly.
- Place the appropriate marker.
- This is figured on the second line under the skull on your Supertech.

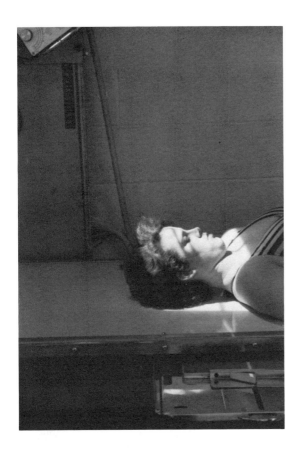

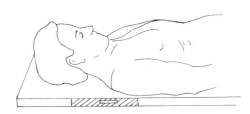

continued

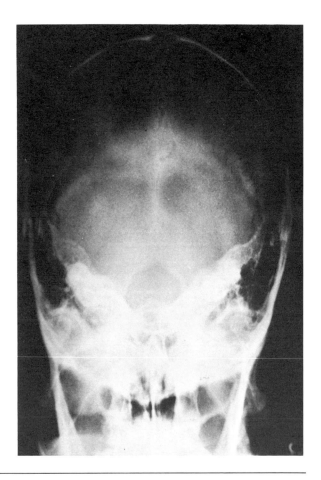

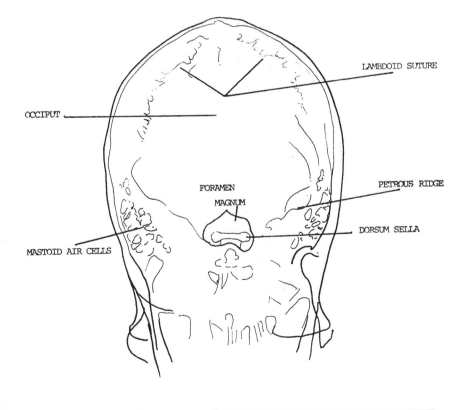

Lateral Skull

Both right and left are included in a series.

Grid   84 to 90 kVp (optimum)
40" SID (FFD)   10 × 12 crosswise

- Patient is prone. Head is turned so the lateral surface is resting on the table.
- *The sagittal plane should be parallel to the film.*
- Central ray is approximately 1 inch above the mid-point of the canthomeatal line.
- Collimate to a little less than film size.
- Measure through the central ray.
- Place the appropriate marker.
- If using a Supertech, this is figured on the first line (under skull).

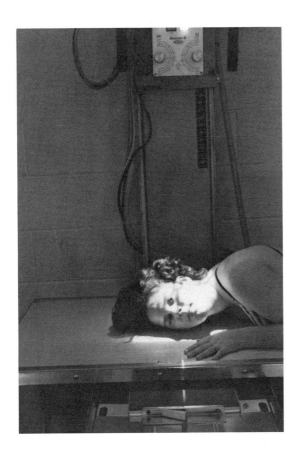

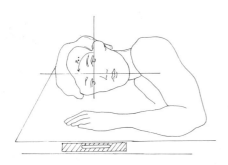

continued

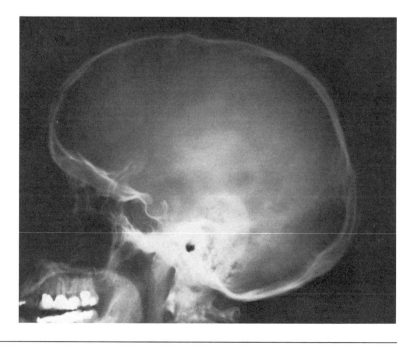

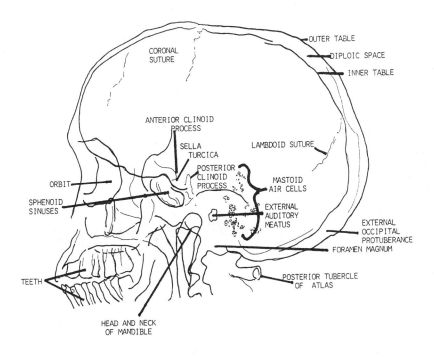

Lateral Skull

Axial View of Skull

Base-Vertex, Submento-Vertex

Grid 84 to 90 kVp
40" SID (FFD) 10 × 12

- Patient is seated or standing. Patient faces tube and extends neck to place top of head against the grid cabinet. The patient's canthomeatal line should be parallel to the cassette.
- The central ray is at the intersection of the sagittal plane with the mid-point of the canthomeatal line. It is directed to enter submentally in the midsagittal plane, pass through the sella turcica, and exit at the vertex of the skull.
- Collimate to a little less than film size.
- Place the appropriate marker.
- If the patient cannot extend the neck sufficiently, a tube tilt may be required to have the central ray pass through the same plane.
- This view is also figured on the second line of your Supertech.

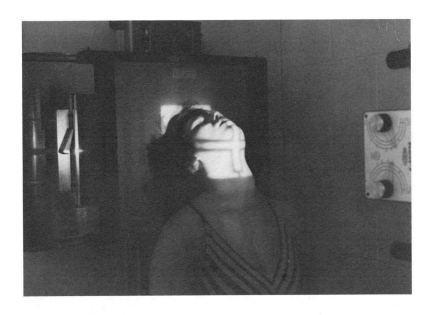

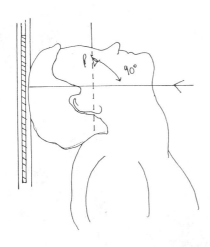

continued

Axial View of Skull: Base-Vertex, Submento-Vertex

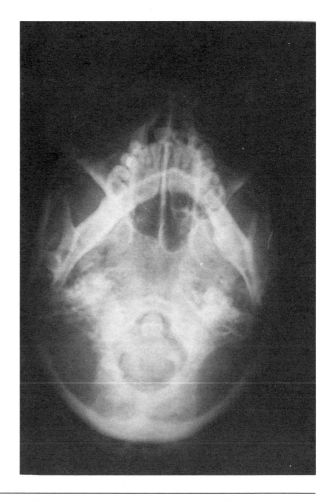

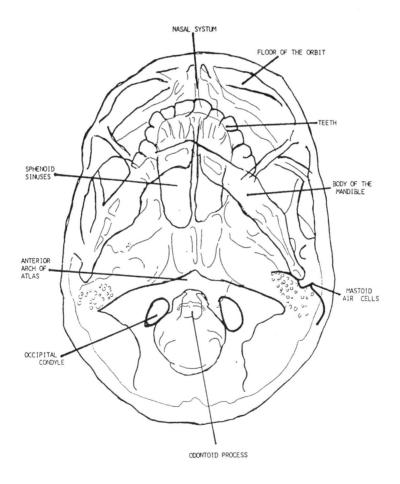

Axial View of Skull: Base-Vertex, Submento-Vertex

Sinuses

Caldwell's Projection
  Posteroanterior
Posteroanterior Water's
Lateral Sinus

Views can be done upright or recumbent. However, at least one view should be done upright.

Caldwell's Projection

Posteroanterior

Grid
40″ SID (FFD)
15 degree caudal tube tilt

80 kVp (optimum)
8 × 10

- Patient is standing, sitting, or recumbent. Position the patient's head so the canthomeatal line is perpendicular to the grid cabinet.
- The central ray is angled 15 degrees caudally and exits at the glabella—the bony prominence in the frontal bone joining the supraorbital ridges.
- Collimate to a little less than film size.
- Measure on the angle of the central ray.
- Place the appropriate marker.

Posteroanterior Water's

Grid
40″ SID (FFD)

84 kVp (optimum)
8 × 10

- Patient is standing, sitting, or recumbent. Place the tip of the patient's chin so that the nose is approximately 1 inch away from the grid cabinet, not resting on the film, and the sagittal plane is perpendicular to the film.
- The central ray enters in the midline and exits 1 inch below the orbits.
- Collimate to a little less than film size.
- Measure through the central ray.
- Place the appropriate marker.

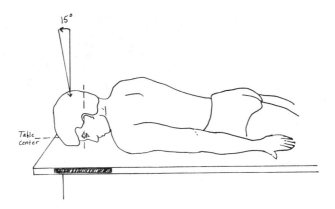

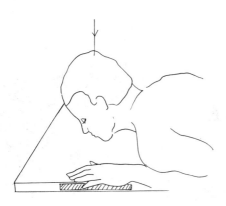

Posteroanterior Water's   215

Lateral Sinus

Grid
40″ SID (FFD)
84 kVp (optimum)
8 × 10

- Patient is either standing, sitting, or recumbent. Place the affected sinus down, so the lateral surface of the head is resting against the table/grid cabinet (true lateral position).
- The central ray should pass through the outer canthus.
- Collimate to a little less than film size.
- Measure through the central ray.
- Place the appropriate marker.
- Be sure there is no tilt or rotation to the head when positioning the patient.
- If using Supertech, add a plus 1½ to the machine correction factor when doing a sinus series.

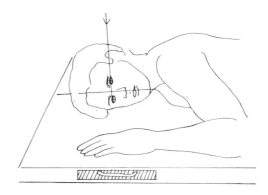

Ribs

Anterior or Posterior Complaints
Oblique Ribs
Tangential Ribs

Whenever possible, do rib studies upright so the patient is not lying on the affected area. A PA chest should be included as part of the rib series to rule out pneumothorax or lung involvement.

Suggested views for a rib series are:

Anterior Complaint
- PA chest
- PA ribs
- 45 degree PA obliques
- Tangential

Posterior Complaint
- PA chest
- AP ribs
- 45 degree AP obliques
- Tangential

Anterior or Posterior Complaints

An AP or PA is performed depending on the area of complaint. Place that portion of the patient closest to the film.

Grid　　　　　　　　　　　80 kVp (optimum)
40" SID (FFD)　　　　　　14 × 17 film

- If the projection is to be below the diaphragm, place the film crosswise.
- The patient is either A to P or P to A. For visualization of the ribs above the diaphragm (1st to 8th), place the cassette 1 inch above C-7 and take the film on full inspiration.
- For visualization of the ribs below the diaphragm (8th to 12th), place the cassette so the bottom of the cassette is at the level of the top of the iliac crests. Take the film on full expiration.
- Measure through the central ray.
- Place the appropriate marker.
- If using a Supertech, be sure to use the proper line on your Supertech—BD is below the diaphragm; AD is above the diaphragm.
- Breathing instructions are given to allow better visualization. Full inspiration lowers the diaphragm; full expiration raises the diaphragm.

Oblique Ribs

Grid
40" SID (FFD)
80 kVp (optimum)
14 × 17 film

In the anterior area of complaint, place the patient P to A.

- Rotate the patient 45 degrees with the affected side closest to the film.
- Rotate the patient 45 degrees with the affected side being brought away from the film.

In the posterior area of complaint, place the patient A to P.

- Rotate the patient 45 degrees with the affected side closest to the film.
- Rotate the patient 45 degrees with the affected side being brought away from the film.

The ribs on the side closest to the film will appear elongated; those brought away from the film will appear shortened.

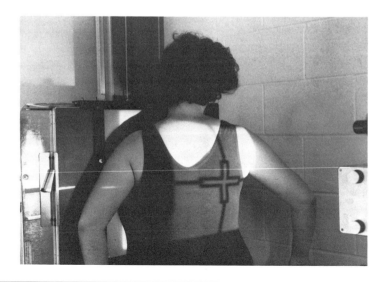

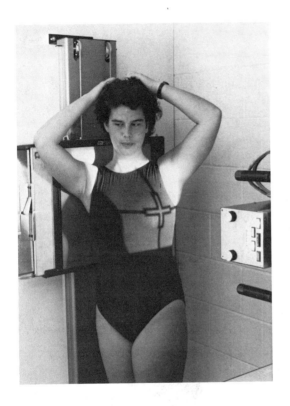

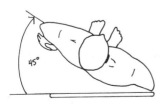
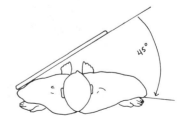

Oblique Ribs

Tangential Ribs

Grid
40″ SID (FFD)
70 kVp (optimum)
10 × 12 lengthwise

- The patient is positioned obliquely with the area of complaint parallel with the central ray (this area is at the most lateral aspect).
- The central ray is directly parallel with the suspected area of rib involvement.
- Measure through the central ray.
- Place the appropriate marker.

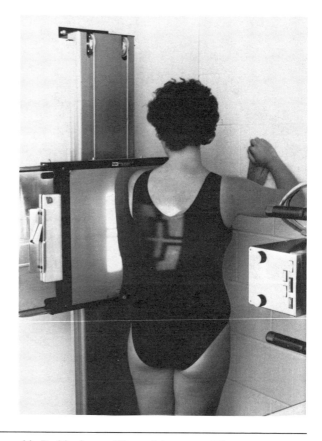

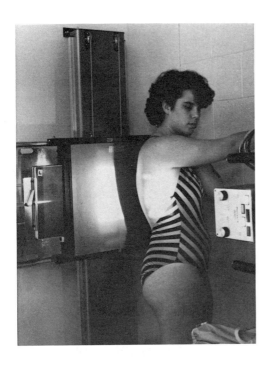

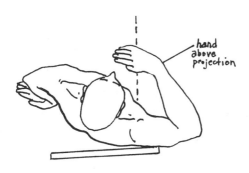

Tangential Ribs 223

Chest

Posteroanterior Chest
Lateral Chest
Apical Lordotic
Full Chest Lordotic

Posteroanterior Chest

Non-Grid (chest plate holder) 100 to 110 kVp (optimum)
72" SID (FFD) 14 × 17 film

- A time of one-tenth of a second or less should be used. If the patient is short and stocky in build, place the 14 × 17 cassette crosswise.
- Patient is standing with back to the tube. The cassette is placed about 2 inches above the patient's shoulders. The patient's chin should be resting on the top of the cassette holder (slightly extended). The arms are rotated and brought out away from the cassette.
- The central ray is at approximately T-6.
- Collimate to a little less than film size.
- Measure over the shoulder, sternum to spine on full inspiration.
- Place the appropriate marker.

This view is done on full inspiration.

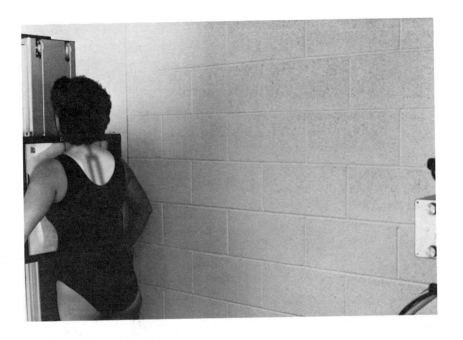

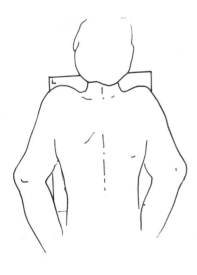

continued

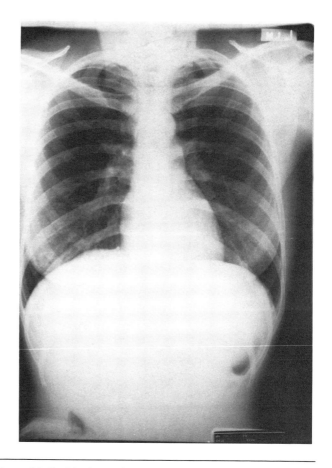

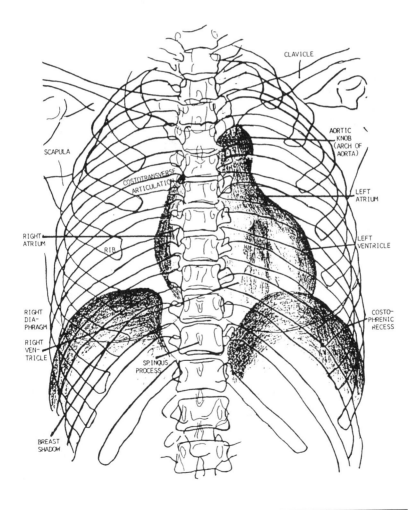

Lateral Chest

Non-Grid (chest plate holder)   100 to 110 kVp (optimum)
72" SID (FFD)   14 × 17 film

- The patient is standing with the left side closest to the cassette. The patient's arms are crossed over the head. The cassette need not be altered from the PA position. Center the patient to the cassette, making sure all the structures are included.
- The central ray is in the axillary region.
- Collimate to a little less than film size.
- Measure the patient at the axillary region on full inspiration.
- Place the appropriate marker.

This view is done on full inspiration.

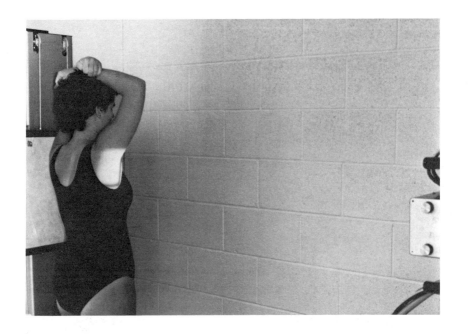

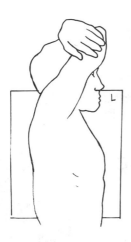

continued

Lateral Chest   231

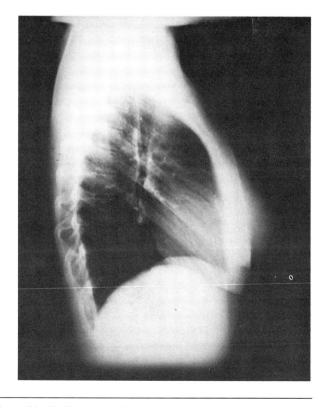

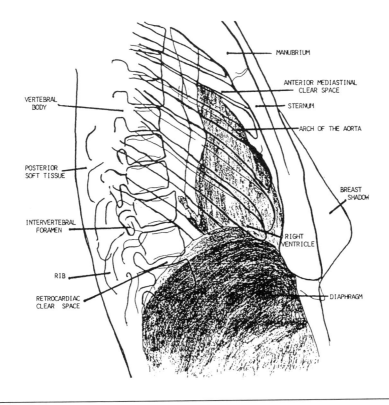

Apical Lordotic

This projection is taken to better visualize the apices of the lungs.

Non-Grid (chest plate holder) 100 to 110 kVp (optimum)
72" SID (FFD) 10 × 12 crosswise
35 degree cephalic tube tilt

- Patient is standing facing the tube (A to P position).
- The central ray is angled 35 degrees cephalad and enters at the center of the body of the sternum. Place the cassette accordingly in line with the angle of the ray.
- Collimate to a little less than film size.
- Measure on the angle of the central ray.
- Place the appropriate marker.

This view is taken on full inspiration.

Full Chest Lordotic

This view is done to better visualize the apices, the right middle lobe, and the lingular area.

- A 14 × 17 film size is used. Positioning and tube tilt are the same as in the apical lordotic view.
- Collimate to a little less than film size.
- Measure on the angle of the ray.
- Place the appropriate marker.

This view is taken on full inspiration.

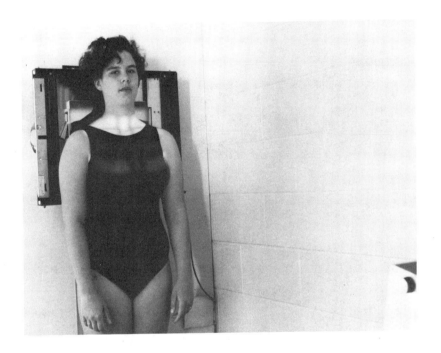

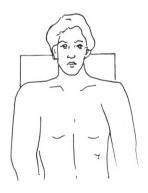

Abdomen

Posteroanterior Abdomen
Kidney, Ureter, Bladder (KUB)
Optional Lateral Abdomen

It is frequently beneficial to do the AP projection upright to visualize and evaluate the movement of viscera. The addition of a PA chest film is recommended when ruling out obstruction or free air.

Posteroanterior Abdomen

Grid
40″ SID (FFD)

100 to 110 kVp (optimum)
14 × 17 film size

- The patient is prone.
- The central ray is midline, 1½ to 2 inches above the iliac crest.
- Collimate to film size.
- Measure through the central ray.
- Place the appropriate marker.

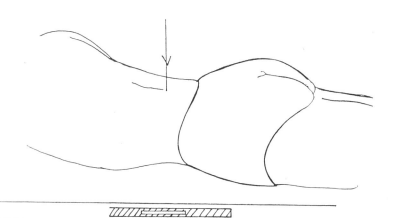

Kidney, Ureter, Bladder (KUB)

Grid
40" SID (FFD)
70 kVp (optimum)
14 × 17 film

- The patient is supine or upright.
- The central ray is midline, at the level of the iliac crests.
- Collimate to a little less than film size.
- Measure through the central ray.
- Place the appropriate marker.

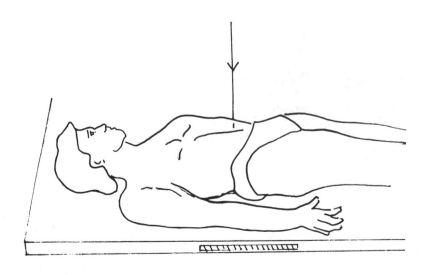

Optional Lateral Abdomen

Grid
40″ SID (FFD)

100 to 110 kVp
14 × 17 or 17 × 14

- The patient is standing or recumbent. He or she is positioned so that a point midway between the anterior and posterior margins of the abdomen is centered to the midline of the table. The knees may be flexed to help stabilize the patient. The arms are raised so that they are not overlying the area to be visualized.
- The central ray is at the level of the iliac crest, however, it may be higher or lower depending on the area of interest and size of abdomen.
- Collimate to a little less than film size.
- Measure through the central ray.
- Place the appropriate marker.

Note. The spine should be included to aid in locating the problem area. If the patient is large it may be necessary to turn the cassette crosswise. The central ray will be more anterior to the spine.

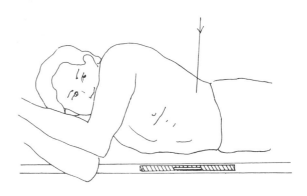

BIBLIOGRAPHY

Bushong SC: Radiologic Science for Technologists. St. Louis, CV Mosby, 1984.

Curry TS, Dowdey JF, Murry RC: Christensen's Introduction to Physics of Diagnostic Radiology. Philadelphia, Lea and Febeger, 1984.

Greenfield GB, Cooper SJ: A Manual of Radiographic Positioning. Philadelphia, JB Lippincott, 1973.

Jacobi CA, Paris DQ: Textbook of Radiologic Technology. St. Louis, CV Mosby, 1977.

Jaeger SA: Radiographic Positioning. Los Angeles, Delta Tau Alpha Fraternity, 1980.

Krakos GT: A look at rare-earth imaging for today's chiropractor. In The Focal Spot. Newsletter of The Council on Diagnostic Imaging, 3:1987.

Meschan I: Synopsis of Radiographic Anatomy. Philadelphia, WB Saunders, 1978.

National Council on Radiation Protection and Measurements: Medical x-ray and gamma-ray protection for energies up to 10 MeV. NCRP 33, Washington DC, NCRP Publications, 1973.

Wicke L: Atlas of Radiologic Anatomy. Baltimore, Urban and Schwarzenberg, 1987.

2
Developmental Variants

Cervical Spine
Ribs
Clavicle
Thoracic Spine
Chest
Lumbar Spine
Pelvis
Upper Extremity
Lower Extremity

Cervical Spine

Block Vertebrae (Failure of Segmentation)
Klippel-Feil Syndrome
Sprengel's Deformity
Hemivertebra
Spina Bifida
Absent Pedicle
Agenesis/Hypoplasia
Odontoid Abnormalities
Ossiculum Terminale Persistens
Occipitalization
Anomalous Articulations
Paramastoid Process
Intercalary Bones
Anterior Tubercle
Posterior Ponticle (Ponticulus Posticus)
Nuchal Bones
Physiological Calcification
Long Styloid Processes
Cervical Ribs

Block Vertebrae (Failure of Segmentation)

Failure of segmentation occurs when segmentation of the somites is disturbed. This can occur at any level and may involve the body, the arch, or the entire segment. When there is a union of the arches, the intervertebral foramen remains sufficiently wide for the exit of the nerves and vessels. These may be flat, round, or oval. Partial union is sometimes associated with a scoliosis.

The congenital block may need to be differentiated from the acquired fusion due to infection, arthritic involvement, or trauma. The total height of a congenital block vertebra is equivalent to the height of the two separate vertebra plus the disc. There is often an indentation, known as a "wasp waist," at the site of the absent disc. A posterior concavity is considered a diagnostic sign of failure of segmentation. In the cervical spine, absence of osteophyte formation at the uncovertebral joints is also indicative of a developmental anomaly.

Early degenerative changes may be noted involving the discs above and below the block vertebra. Intervertebral foramina alterations may also occur due to increased stress on the adjacent joints, as they attempt to take over the function of the fixed vertebra.

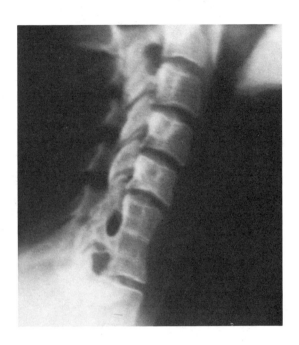

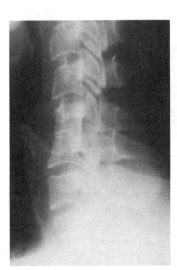

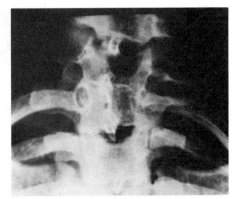

Rudimentary disc spaces and "wasp waist" indentations at the site of the disc space.
continued

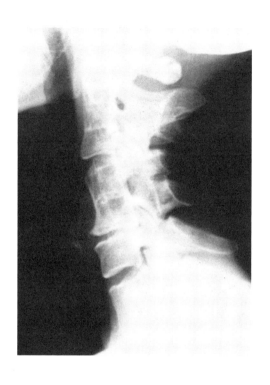

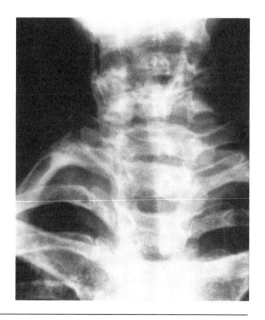

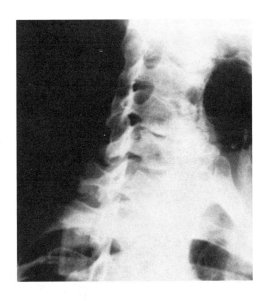

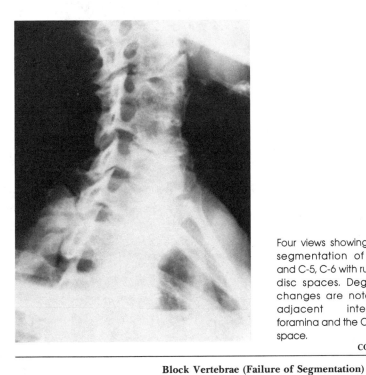

Four views showing failure of segmentation of C-2–C-4, and C-5, C-6 with rudimentary disc spaces. Degenerative changes are noted of the adjacent intervertebral foramina and the C-6–C7 disc space.

continued

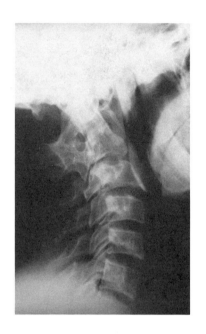

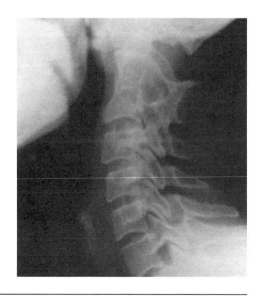

Two views showing C-2, C-3 failure of segmentation with possible occipitalization atlas anomalies.

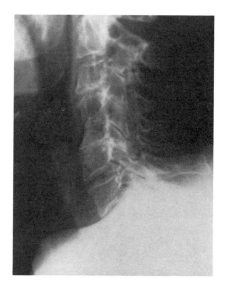

C-4, C-5 failure of segmentation with marked degenerative changes noted above and below.

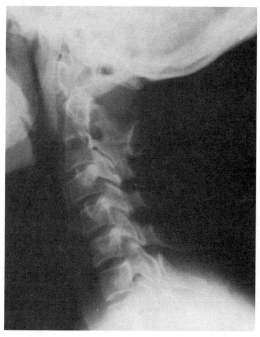

C-2, C-3 congenital block vertebra.

continued

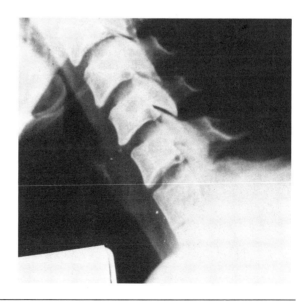

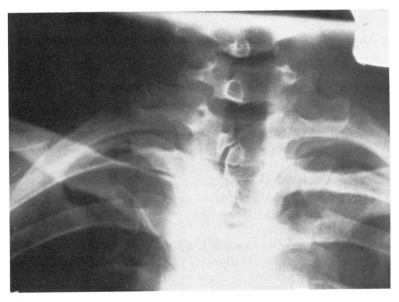
Two views showing C-7–T-1 failure of segmentation with rudimentary disc space.

Klippel-Feil Syndrome

Klippel-Feil syndrome was first described in 1912 as a combination of congenital malformations involving the lower cervical spine, extensive fusions, marked shortening of the neck, and often a rounded back. The three clinical signs that must be present are a short neck, low posterior hairline, and limited range of motion. The block vertebrae may involve the neural arch. The intervertebral foramina are then often smaller, smooth, round, or oval with a large spinous process. Flattening and widening of the involved bodies may be demonstrated. Hemivertebrae, spina bifida occulta, and absence of hypoplasia of one or more discs and other anomalies may also be noted. A variety of problems may be associated with this syndrome, such as torticollis, facial asymmetry, widening of the neck, and difficulty in breathing or swallowing. Neurologic manifestations vary—spasticity, hyperreflexia, pain, muscle atrophy, oculomotor disturbances, pyramidal tract findings, paralysis, anesthesia, and paresthesia have been experienced. When high fusions (upper cervical segments) are present, the neurologic symptoms tend to be more prominent and appear earlier.

Scoliosis of 20 degrees or more is found in over half the cases. Sprengel's deformity is present in over one-fifth of the cases, especially those with high and extensive block vertebra. In as many as two-thirds of the cases GU symptoms are encountered. These symptoms may include unilateral renal agenesis, kidney malrotation, double collecting systems, renal ectopia, bicornuate uterus with vaginal agenesis, penis and testicular abnormalities, and urethral duplications. Various types of hearing impairments (conductive, sensory-neural, and mixed) have been found in approximately one-third of the cases and absence of the external auditory meatus has been reported. Cardiac abnormalities and mental deficiencies have also been noted in this syndrome.

Upper thoracic segments may be affected in the failure of segmentation along with other developmental defects. Hypermobility of the unfused segments often leads to early degenerative joint disease.

Although the exact cause is unknown, it has been attributed to intrauterine inflammations or fusions (Bassoe). It should be remembered that not all segmentation defects in the cervical spine are a part of this syndrome.

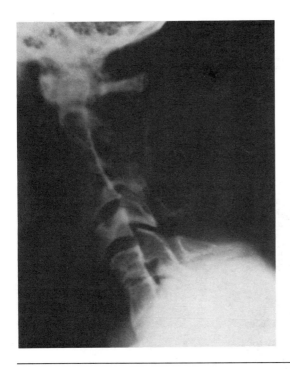

Klippel-Feil syndrome—failure of segmentation noted at C-2–C-4 and C-6–T-1.

Sprengel's Deformity

Sprengel's deformity is a congenital anomaly in which the scapula fails to descend normally. The position of the scapula is so that the superior angle lies in a plane higher than the neck of the first rib. It is usually medially rotated so the inferior angle points toward the spine. The scapula may be normal in shape or there may be a decrease in its vertical diameter and increased width. It is often smaller in size. The finding usually is unilateral, but may be bilateral. It is seen in association with Klippel-Feil syndrome 25% to 30% of the time.

In approximately 30% to 40% of cases, a connection is noted between the elevated scapula and one of the vertebra, usually the fifth or sixth cervical. This may be an osseous, cartilaginous, or fibrous union, and is called an omovertebral or suprascapular bone.

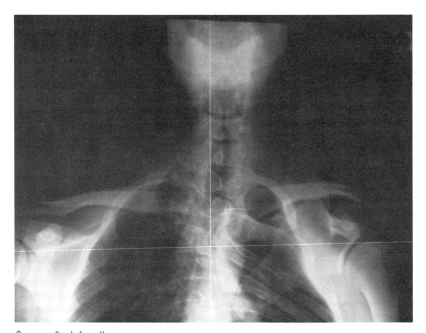

Sprengel's deformity.

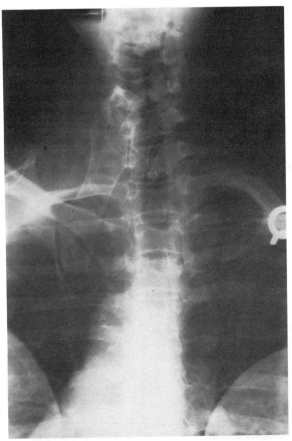

Sprengel's deformity with an omovertebral bone.

Hemivertebra

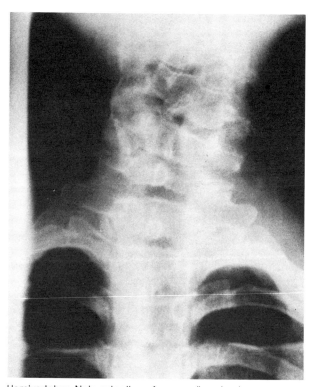

Hemivertebra. Note adaption of surrounding structures.

Spina Bifida

In the cervical region, the first, second, and seventh segments are the most often affected with spina bifida. In fact, posterior spina bifida of the atlas is the most common C-1 malformation and according to Geipel occurs in about 3 % of the population. Spina bifida of the ring of C-1 is almost always without complications. Asymmetry of the articular processes between C-1 and C-2 has been associated. Anterior spina bifida is a rather infrequent finding.

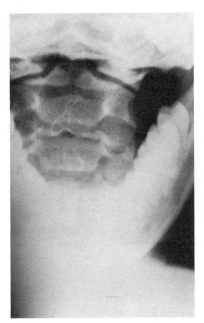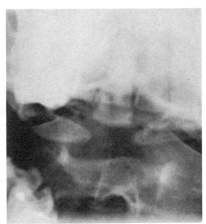

Spina bifida of the posterior arch of the atlas. Note the variation in the size of the cleft (two views) *continued.*

continued

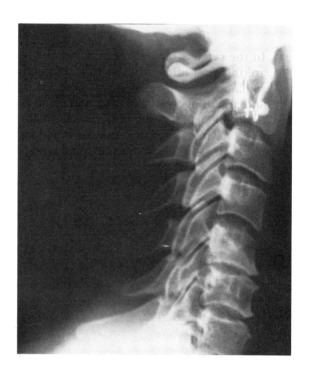

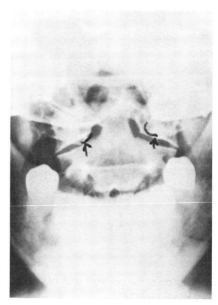

Spina bifida of the posterior arch of the atlas. Note the variation in the size of the cleft (two views).

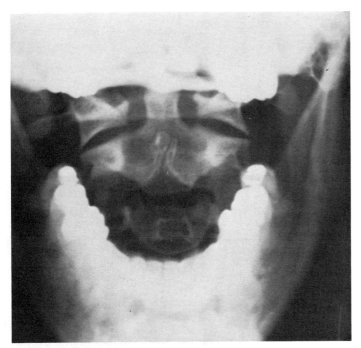

C-2 spina bifida occulta.

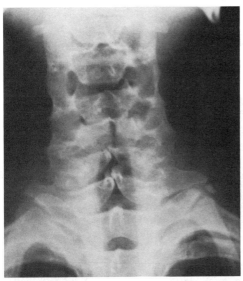

C-6, C-7 spina bifida occulta. Persistent first rib apophysis.

continued

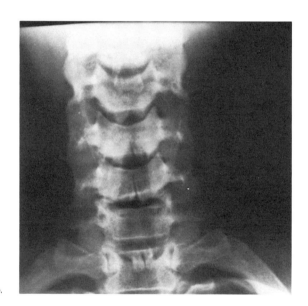

Spina bifida occulta C-6.

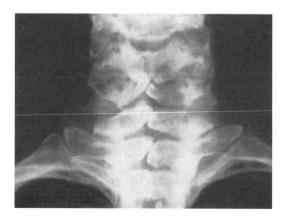

Spina bifida occulta of C-6–T-1.

Absent Pedicle

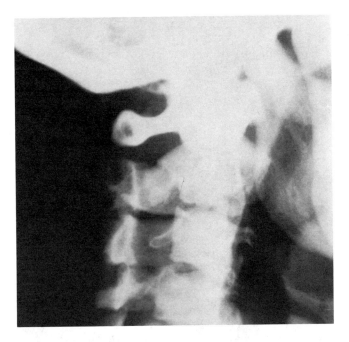

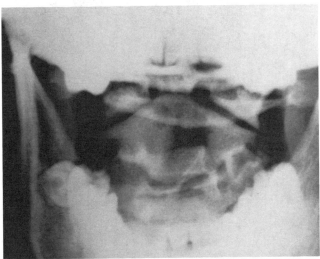

Absent pedicle due to failure of osseous formation. While not clinically significant these must be differentiated from erosion due to a dumbbell-type intraspinal tumor or tortuous or aneurysmal vertebral artery. In the thoracic and lumbar spine the main differentials are malignancy and inflammatory disease.

Agenesis/Hypoplasia

Agenesis or hypoplasia of varying degrees is a common condition. This may be encountered at any level of the spine, however, it frequently occurs at the transition levels.

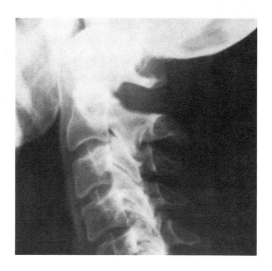

Hypoplasia of the posterior tubercle of the atlas.

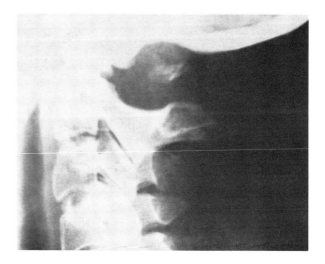

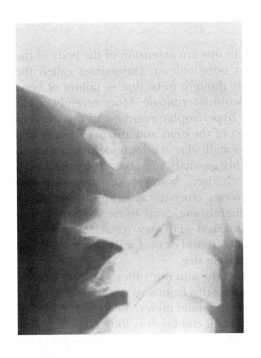

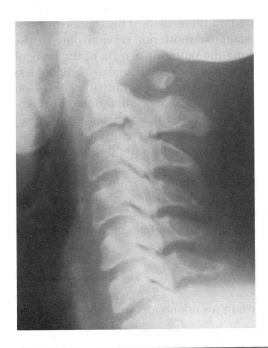

Agenesis (more accurately called failure of ossification) of the posterior arch of the atlas. This is usually not significant, however, cases of instability have been reported. (three views).

Odontoid Abnormalities

The odontoid process is an upward extension of the body of the second vertebra. The os odontoideum (sometimes called the "third condyle") is usually thought to be due to failure of bony union of the normal ossiculum terminale. More recently, it has been considered a large hypertrophic remnant of the proatlas associated with hypoplasia of the dens and absence of the distal ossification center. Occasionally the os odontoideum attaches to the arch of the atlas. This anomaly may be an asymptomatic condition even in active children, however, in later years with ligamentous (e.g., transverse, cruciate, alar, apical dental ligaments, and tentorial membrane) and muscular laxity, the instability may become marked and may result in cord compression. The ossicle may be round or oval with a smooth, dense border and may be of variable size.

Should hypertrophy of the anterior tubercle of the atlas be noted, it helps to differentiate this from a recent fracture. It does not rule out the possibility of an old injury. The enlargement of the tubercle indicates that the condition is long standing. Forward and backward gliding motion may be demonstrated radiographically. Flexion and extension should be conducted voluntarily by the patient. The sagittal diameter of the spinal canal should be evaluated on these views. This is done by measuring from the spino-laminar (posterior cervical) line of the atlas to a line drawn along the posterior margin of the body of the axis. Generally, reduction of the spinal canal to 13 mm or less or excessive instability, greater than 10 mm translation of C-1 on 2 through the complete range of motion (determined by subtracting the spinal canal diameter on flexion from its measurement on extension) may be associated with neurologic problems. Rarely do these patients have symptoms referable to the cranial nerves.

Trivial cervical trauma may result in serious neurologic disability. Other anomalies, such as basilar invagination, have been noted to occur with this anomaly.

Schiller and Nieda classified malformations of the odontoid process as

1. Complete absence
2. Partial absence
3. Separation or nonfusion (os odontoideum)

It was their opinion that all three of these forms led to an unstable atlanto-axial joint with potential pressure on the cervical cord or medulla.

It must be recalled that the apex and base of odontoid process fuse at approximately 9 years of age, but that the base does not fuse to the body of C-2 until adulthood. This situation is normal and must not be construed as an os odontoideum unless the odontoid is displaced.

Prophylactic stabilization is still controversial in the asymptomatic patient. Surgical intervention is frequent in unstable cases or with severe neurological manifestation. Presenting symptoms may be headaches, transient paresis, neck pain, ataxia, intermittent loss of consciousness, or suspected cerebral palsy.

continued

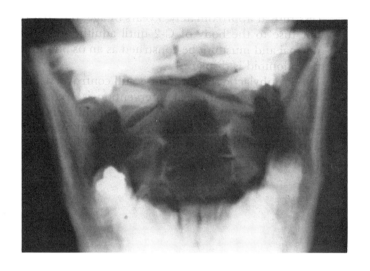

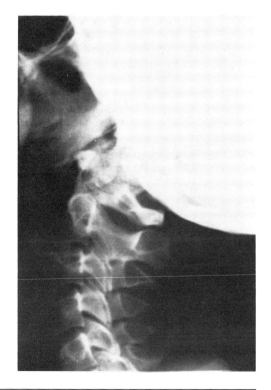

Os odontoideum. Note ossicle above base on tomogram (two views).

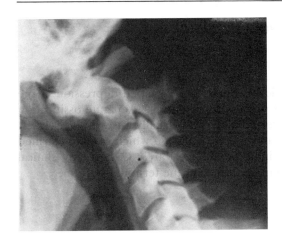

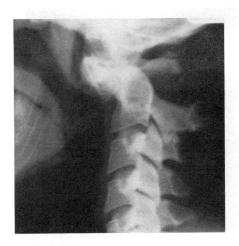

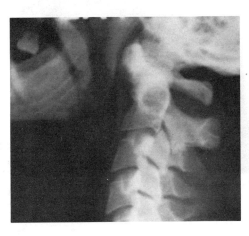

Os odontoideum. Note gliding on the flexion and extension views. Patient had no neurological symptoms (three views).

Ossiculum Terminale Persistens

Ossiculum terminale persistens is a v-shaped depression at the tip of the odontoid process representing a separate ossification center (ossiculum terminale). This usually fuses by age 12. It may never be present or may persist, in which case it is termed the ossiculum terminale persistens. Rarely is there any clinical significance of anomalies affecting the terminal portion.

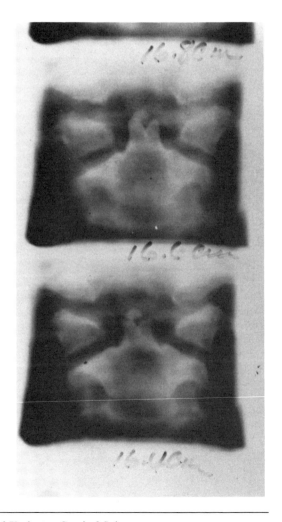

Occipitalization

Occipitalization of the atlas implies fusion of all, or portions, of the atlas to the base of the skull. This may be associated with basilar invagination, dysplasia of the odontoid process, platybasia, or deformity of the foramen magnum (decrease in size and irregular in shape). The diagnosis of this cannot be made clinically, but must be demonstrated radiographically by flexion and extension views showing absence of motion between the atlanto-occipital joint. Tomography is often necessary to confirm this. Symptoms are not always present. Neurologic findings are typically not manifested until later in adolescence or adulthood. In approximately one-half of the cases synostosis of C-2 and C-3 is also present.

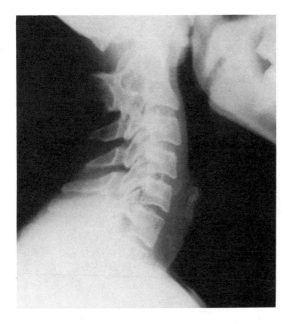

Assimilation of the atlas and C-2, C-3 failure of segmentation.

Anomalous Articulations

Anomalous articulations may occur at any level. They are usually only significant if they alter normal biomechanics, however, it is possible that a bursa or degenerative changes may develop, in which case symptomatology may then be present.

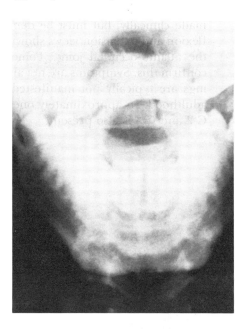

Anomalous C-1 — C-2 articulation.

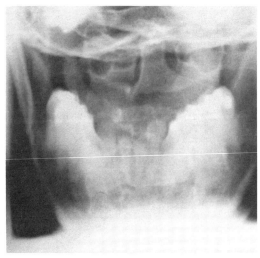

Anomalous articulation between atlas and axis (right angle joint configuration).

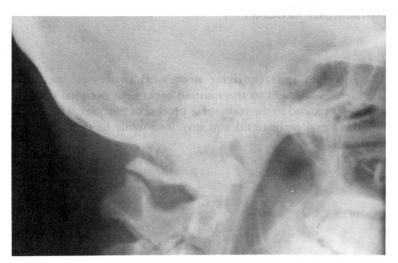

Anomalous articulation between the posterior tubercle of the atlas and the spinous process of C-2.

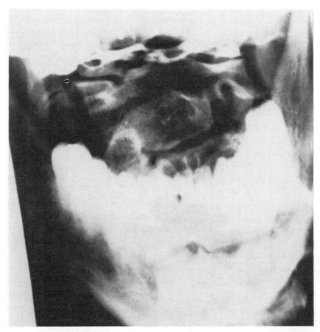

Reversed angulation of the lateral mass and axis articulation. Also note apparent "stubby" odontoid process and a paramastoid process.

Anomalous Articulations

Paramastoid Process

Paramastoid (paracondylar processes) processes are bony eminences adjacent to the mastoid process or occipital condyle that may extend to the transverse process of the atlas. These may be unilateral or bilateral and are not usually of clinical significance.

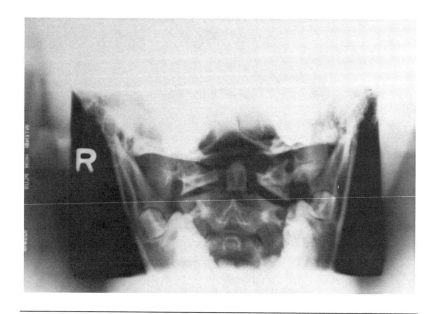

Intercalary Bones

Intercalary bones are small bony ossicles in the anterior vertebral interspaces, usually in the cervical spine. Various theories have been expressed as to their origin, including ununited ossification centers, calcification in the anterior longitudinal ligament, and calcification/ossification of the disc—a precursor of degenerative changes. Most often these are considered to be of little clinical significance.

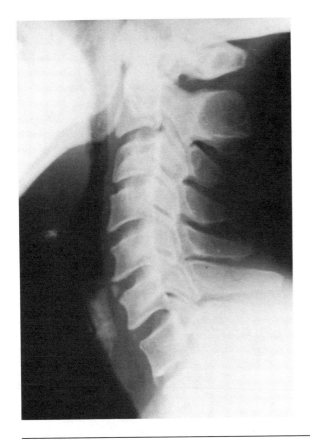

Anterior Tubercle

Elongation of the anterior tubercle of the transverse process of a cervical vertebra appears as a bony mass projecting anterior to the vertebral body on a lateral film. This should not be confused with marked osteophyte formation. Unlike an osteophyte, this arises posterior to the anterior margins of the vertebral body (from the area of the transverse process). The anterior tubercle is another manifestation of a costal component of a cervical vertebra, similar to a cervical rib. It was first identified by Lapayowski in 1912, and is most commonly found on the sixth cervical segment. It is a relatively rare anomaly. Anterior tubercles are often of no clinical importance, but occasionally have symptoms similar to those of a cervical rib, i.e., tingling and weakness in the arm. In cases of trauma they should not be mistaken for a fracture fragment.

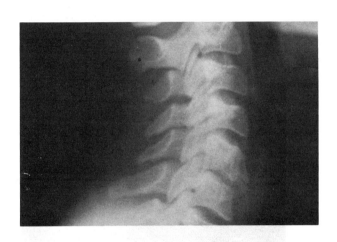

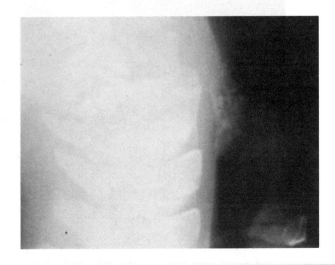

Posterior Ponticle (Ponticulus Posticus)

According to Shinz, 10% of all cervical spine examinations demonstrated this anomaly. It is formed by the ossification of the oblique membrane of the atlanto-occipital ligament. It originates at the posterior margin of the superior articular surface of the atlas and often extends to the upper margin of the posterior arch of the atlas. This forms the arcuate foramen (foramen arcuale) through which usually passes the suboccipital nerve and the vertebral artery.

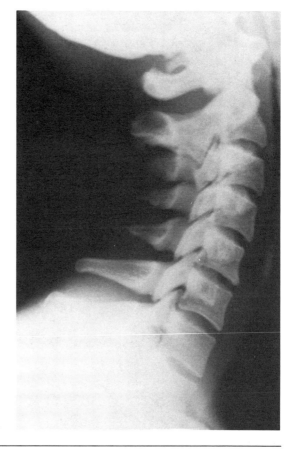

Partial posterior ponticle.

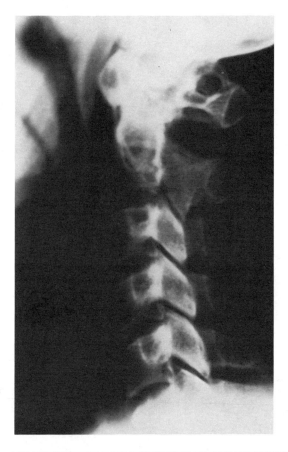

Posterior ponticle. Note double density one on each side of the posterior arch.

Nuchal Bones

Ligamentous calcifications and ossifications are not considered to be clinically significant. Nuchal bones or calcifications/ossifications within the nuchal ligament are not an uncommon finding. These may be in any part of this posterior structure and may vary in number, size, and shape. Periodically, a prominent external occipital protuberance is noted. This may be due to the ossification of the nuchal ligament at its attachment.

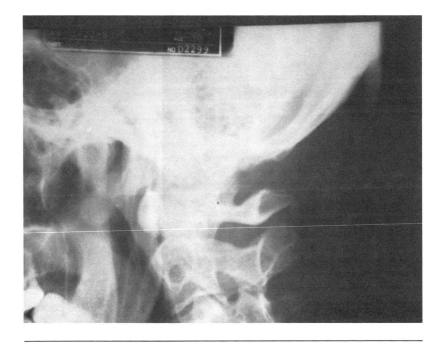

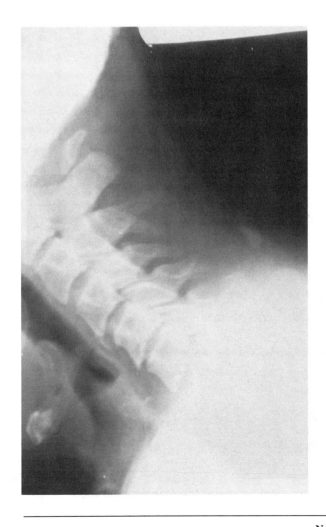

Physiological Calcification

Physiologic calcifications may occur in a variety of structures without clinical importance. This presentation is commonly found in the thyroid cartilage, tracheal rings, pineal gland, and costal cartilage.

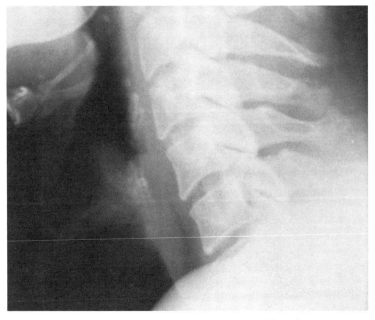

Mottled calcification within the lateral horn of the thyroid cartilage.

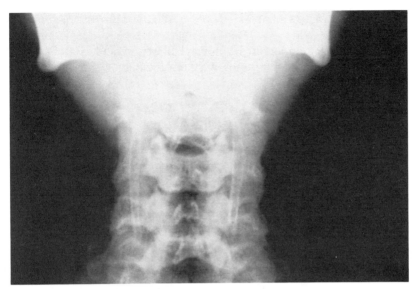

Lateral horn of the thyroid cartilage, calcified, giving the appearance of a "railroad track" across the articular pillar.

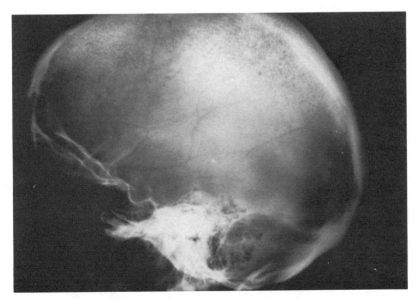

Pineal gland calcification.

Long Styloid Processes

Stylohyoid ligament calcification is common and ordinarily causes no symptoms. Rigidity of an elongated styloid process with any alteration in its normal direction and contour may, however, cause symptoms by compressing on adjacent structures.

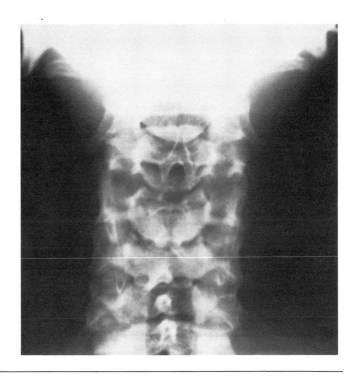

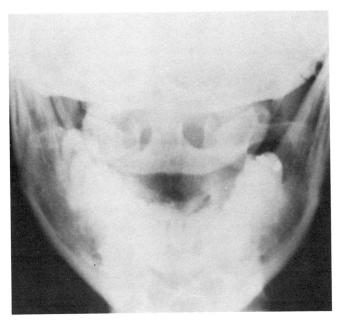

Long styloid processes of the temporal bones. Note long transverse processes of the atlas (two views).

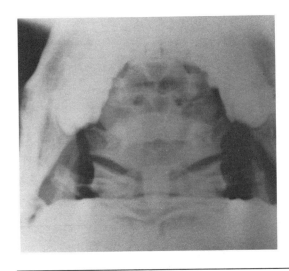

Long styloid processes of the temporal bones.

Cervical Ribs

The cervical section is extremely stable and is considered a constant count of seven. There are some congenital cervico-occipital anomalies that may alter the appearance, but not the count. The presence of a cervical rib does not affect the numbering of the vertebrae. Cervical ribs are felt to occur in .5% to 1% of all humans. They may be either unilateral or bilateral. The majority are bilateral, and usually asymmetrical. They are encountered 10% to 15% more frequently in females. (To aid in differentiating a cervical rib from the first thoracic rib, the orientation of the transverse processes of C-7 is downward or horizontal while the thoracic transverse processes have an upward projection.) When the rib is short or no rib articulation is actually evident, a fibrous band may be present. Articulation or fusion with the first rib may be noted.

Cervical ribs or fibrous bands are often asymptomatic. Symptoms occur in less than 10% of patients and are usually not manifested until middle age. The symptoms may be disabling when they compress subclavian vessels and the brachial plexus. Typical symptoms include pain and weakness of the arm, swelling of the hand, and variations in the intensity of the pulses in certain positions.

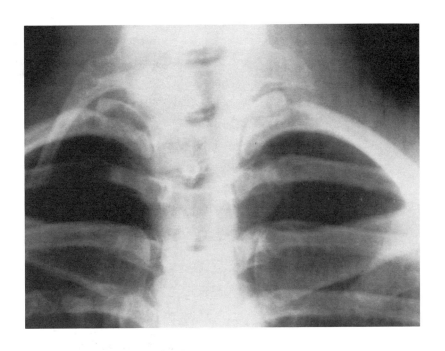

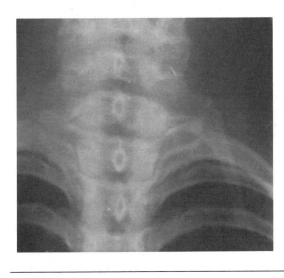

Various presentations of cervical ribs and hyperplastic transverse processes (two views).

continued

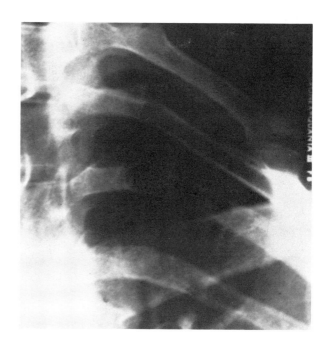
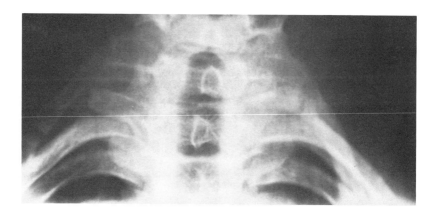

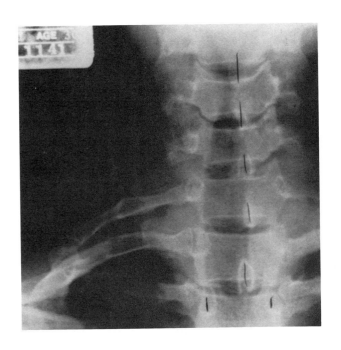

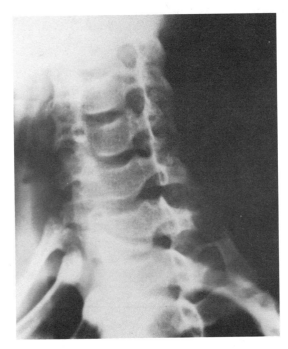

Four presentations of cervical ribs with articulations.

Cervical Ribs

Ribs

Pseudoarthrosis
Intrathoracic
Agenesis
Ectopic
Synostosis
Forked
Costal Cartilage Calcification

Pseudoarthrosis

Pseudoarthrosis of the first rib is possibly a developmental alteration, although, another explanation of this finding is an ununited fracture.

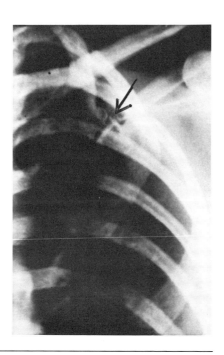

Intrathoracic

Intrathoracic ribs arise within the bony thorax, most often on the right side. They usually arise from the postero-inferior margin of a normal rib or a vertebral body. Frequently they extend downward and slightly lateral, ending at or near the diaphragm. Sometimes these are attached to the diaphragm by a fibrous band.

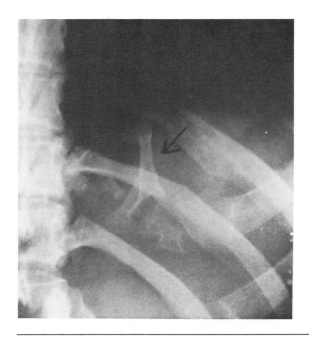

Agenesis

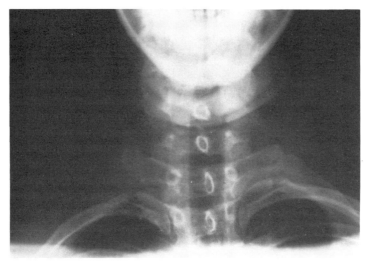

Agenesis of the first rib.

Ectopic

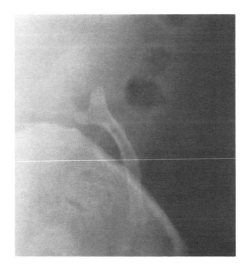

Ectopic rib formation.

Synostosis

Synostosis in females is not an uncommon finding, more often seen on the right involving the first and second ribs. However, any level may be involved and any part affected. The more frequent areas are the lateral portions along the angle and the vertebral ends. Little or no clinical significance is given to this anomaly. The only importance is that it may lead to an erroneous interpretation of an abnormal lung density.

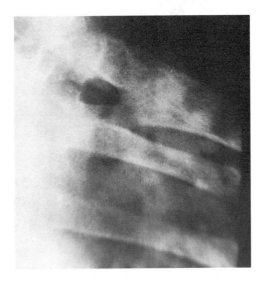

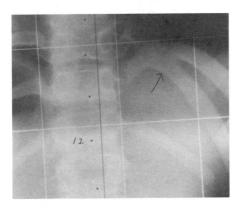

Rib synostosis (two views).

Forked

Forked ribs (also referred to as anterior bifurcation or bifid). This is the second most common rib anomaly following cervical ribs. Most frequent sites are the third and fourth ribs, more commonly on the right. Little or no clinical significance is placed on this finding.

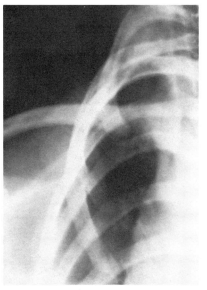

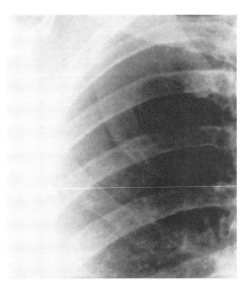

Forked (bifid) ribs (two views).

Costal Cartilage Calcification

Costal cartilage calcification is present to some degree in the majority of the human population by the age of 25. Calcification of the first costal cartilage begins in the early part of the third decade and often precedes calcification of other cartilage. This finding is uncommon in males under the age of 20. It is present in 45.2% of the female population under 20 years of age. Differences in the patterns of calcification have been noted. The upper and lower borders become calcified first in males, creating the "railroad track sign." In females the central portion calcifies first, giving the appearance of a "wagging tongue." These findings have no relationship to any disease. It is felt that it is a physiologic response of the connective tissue to the demands of the muscular activity and reaction to the greater rigidity of the chest wall.

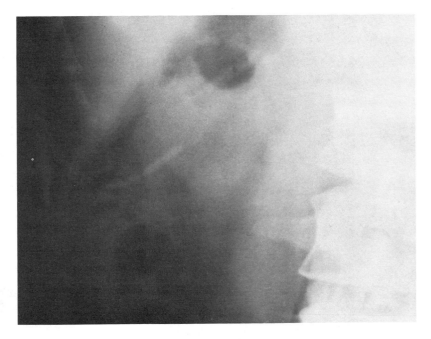

Calcification in the first costal cartilage.

continued

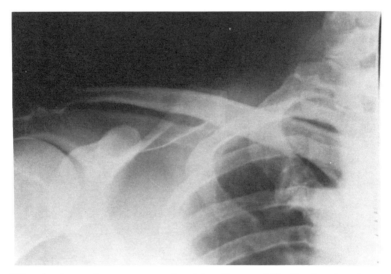

"Wagging tongue" appearance of costal cartilage calcification in a female.

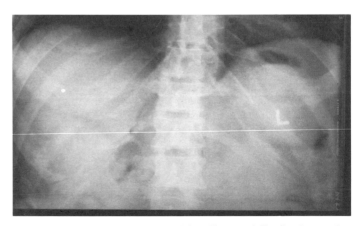

"Railroad track" appearance of costal cartilage calcification in a male.

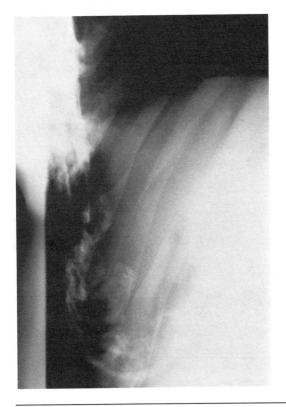

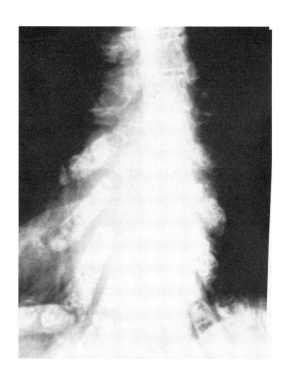

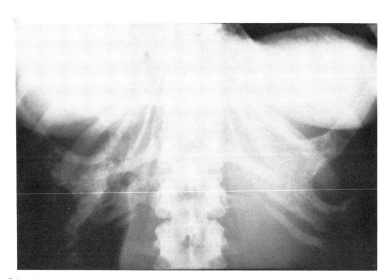

Extensive costal cartilage calcification (three views).

Clavicle

Rhomboid Fossae
Medial Ends
Foramen

Rhomboid Fossae

Rhomboid fossae are normal anatomical structures. They provide attachment to the rhomboid or costoclavicular ligaments that bind the clavicle to the first rib. The fossae are depressions that vary from slight roughening to deep indentations on the inferior surface of the clavicles, 1 to 3 cm from their sternal end. These may be either unilateral or bilateral. They are of no clinical significance and should not be confused with an erosive alteration.

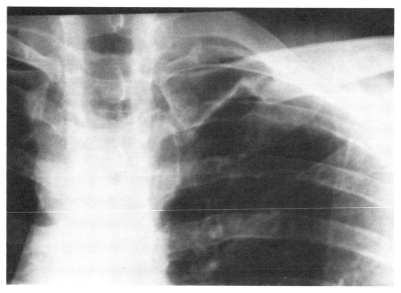

Unilateral rhomboid fossa.

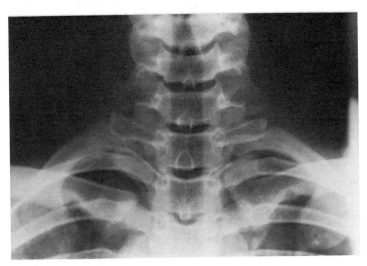

Bilateral rhomboid fossa.

Medial Ends

The medial ends of the clavicle may remain cupped or irregular. Without associated symptoms these should not be mistaken for evidence of inflammatory arthropathy or metabolic bone disorder.

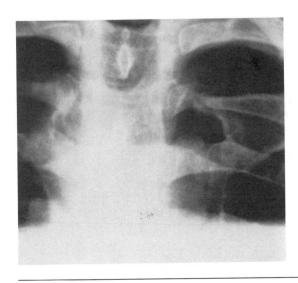

Foramen

A small foramen may occasionally be seen near the center of the clavicle on its superior aspect. This finding may be unilateral or bilateral. This foramen permits the passage of the middle supraclavicular nerve. It is said to be present in 6% of dry skeletal specimens.

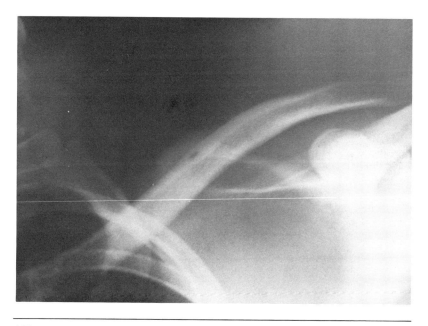

Thoracic Spine

Hahn's Fissures
Hemivertebrae
Persistent Apophyses
Dorsal Hemivertebra

Hahn's Fissures

Hahn's fissures (notches, clefts) are slit-like indentations that run horizontally across the central portion of the vertebral body representing a vascular groove. They are of no clinical significance.

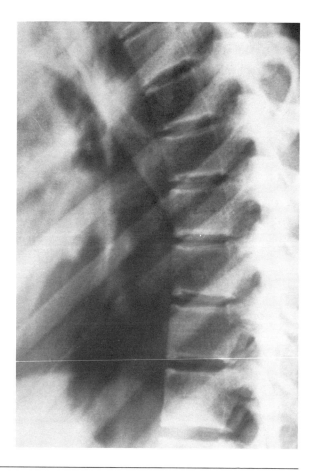

Hemivertebra

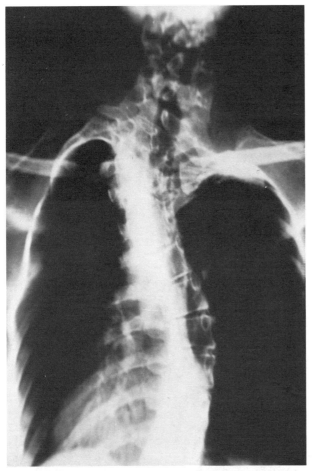

Multiple unbalanced hemivertebrae with a progressive scoliosis. Spina bifida occulta are also noted.

Persistent Apophyses

Typically the apophyses have united by the 21st year. Any secondary center of ossification may persist and are usually only of anatomical interest. When there is a history of trauma, the possibility of fracture may arise. The persistent ossicles most often have smooth cortical margins.

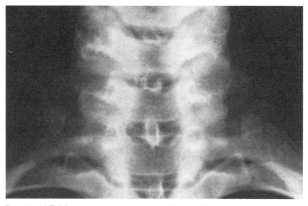

Persistent T-1 transverse process on the right.

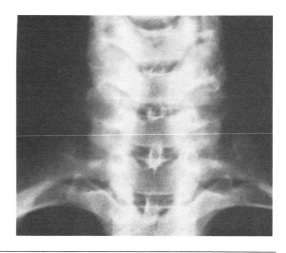

Ununited apophysis of the T-1 transverse process is a relatively frequent finding with no clinical significance.

Dorsal Hemivertebra

Dorsal hemivertebra may simulate a compression fracture and a gibbus deformity may develop. They must be differentiated from the result of trauma or a pathological process such as an infection. With a dorsal hemivertebra all the bones appear healthy, usually the anterior half of the vertebra is absent, not compressed. The adjacent vertebrae are enlarged to fit the deformity. No anterior bulging is present. Other abnormalities in development may be noted. The rib interspaces are normal. When a severe kyphosis develops, late complications such as paraplegia and reduced pulmonary function may result.

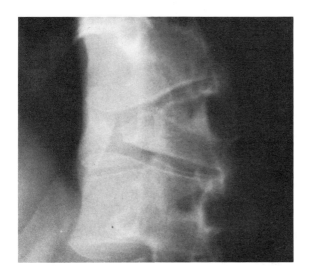

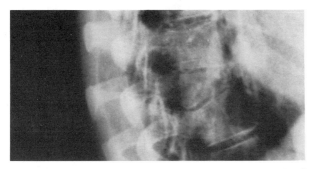

Two examples of dorsal hemivertebra. Note adaptation of adjacent segments.

Chest

Pectus Excavatum (Funnel Chest)
Pectus Carinatum (Pigeon Breast)
Azygos (Azygous) Lobe

Pectus Excavatum (Funnel Chest)

Pectus excavatum (funnel chest) is a depression of the sternum in which the ribs on each side protrude anteriorly more than the sternum itself. This is generally felt to be of genetic origin and is found occasionally in children with heart murmurs. The most frequent murmur simulates pulmonic stenosis, presumably the result of a kinking in the pulmonary artery with increased splitting of the second heart sound. Pathological heart findings have been found, but most of the patients have normal, healthy hearts. Cosmetic reasons are usually the cause for surgical intervention.

On a PA or AP radiograph of the chest, the following findings may be noted:

1. More vertical angulation of the anterior portion of the ribs with the degree of slant roughly proportional to the amount of depression.
2. Displacement of the heart shadow to the left with some convexity of its upper border, so that the appearance of the cardiac silhouette suggests mitral valve disease with enlargement and prominence of the left auricular appendage. On the lateral projection, the sternal indentation is apparent.

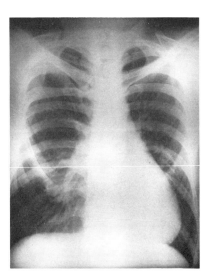
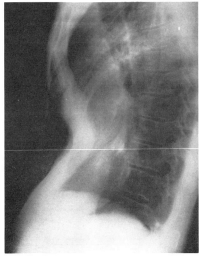

Pectus Carinatum (Pigeon Breast)

Pectus carinatum (pigeon breast) is a congenital or acquired deformity of the sternum with anterior protrusion of the sternum and costal cartilages that develop with growth. This is best seen on the lateral projection. Typically no significant abnormalities are noted on the A to P film. In the congenital variety the majority of patients are asymptomatic, however, it has been stated that those who have this deformity are more prone to respiratory infections. The acquired form is usually associated with atrial or ventricular septal defects or long-term asthmatics.

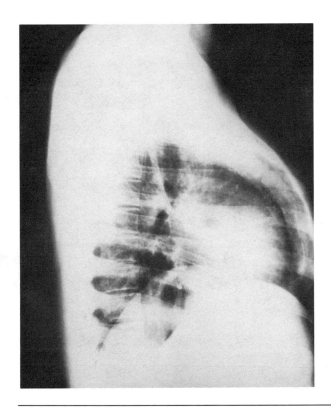

Azygos (Azygous) Lobe

This finding is created by the azygous vein when it fails to migrate medially. A curvilinear shadow that extends obliquely across the upper portion of the right lung is formed by the four pleural layers—two parietal and two visceral. The fissure ends in a "teardrop" or "comma" with its tail pointing upward, caused by the vein itself. This will be found at a variable distance above the right hilum. Felson states that this fissure is visible in .4% of the population. No clinical significance is given to the fissure itself, although, a disease process may occur in the lobe that is formed.

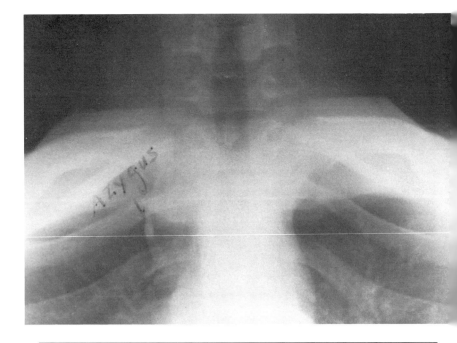

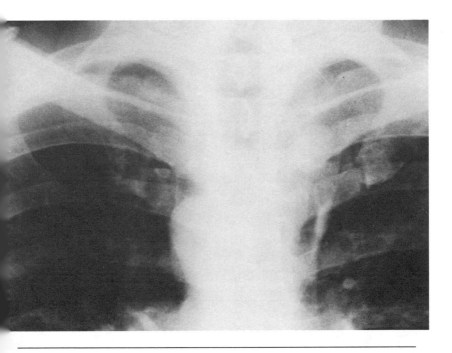

Lumbar Spine

Spina Bifida Occulta
Knife Clasp Deformity
Transitional Segments
Hemivertebrae
Butterfly Vertebra
Failure of Segmentation
Anomalous Articulations
Asymmetrical Facets
Tropism
Hypoplasia/Agenesis
Persistent Secondary Ossification Centers
Limbus Bone
Nuclear Impressions
Iliolumbar Ligament Calcification

Spina Bifida Occulta

Spina bifida occulta (spinal dysraphism) or an ossification defect in the spinous process or lamina occurs in 5% to 10% of the general population. It is common at the lumbosacral region (in approximately 20% in its simplest form) and transitional areas but has been observed at virtually every spinal level. The size of the cleft may vary from a slight midline cleft to absence of most of the vertebral arch. The area is often filled with fibrous tissue and may attach superficially to the skin producing a dimple. At times the cleft may actually be palpated between the two deviating tips of the spinous processes and lamina. Occasionally, an ossicle is noted between the cleft. This probably develops within the ligamentum flavum from a separate center like those on the transverse and spinous processes. In the absence of such a center, the "unclosed" spinal canal is well protected by the dense, tough ligamentum flavum.

Although usually asymptomatic, there may be an associated clue to a more serious neuroanatomic defect. Some are associated with strangling of the nerve roots by fibrous bands and lipomas. Statistically the occurence of spina bifida occulta with spondylolysis and spondylolisthesis is common, however, it is not known if this is coincidental or causal.

Some researchers feel that a spina bifida occulta may predispose patients to disc problems when they suffer injury, while others question whether or not this is an area of localized weakness, lesion, or anomaly. Others deny any relationship to low back pain.

If the arch defect is very wide or noted at multiple levels, a soft tissue mass is present, and there are neurological manifestations; this is then called a spina bifida vera or manifesta.

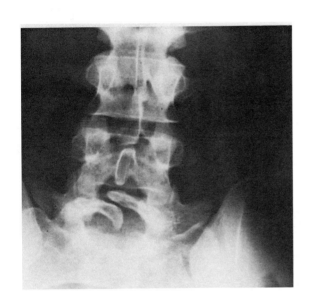

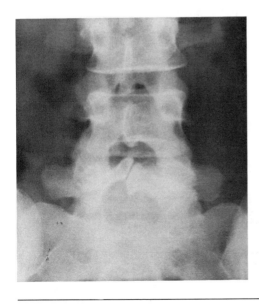

L-5 spina bifida occulta.
continued

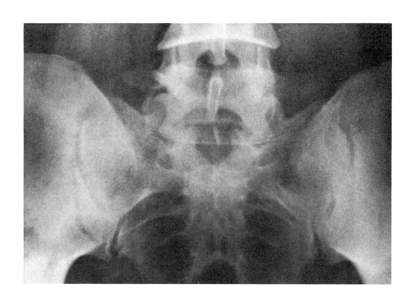

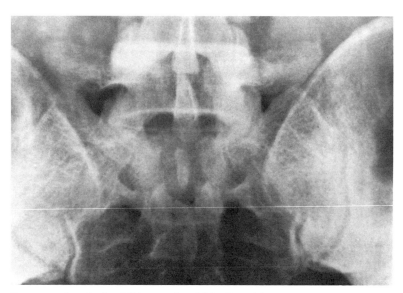

Two examples of spina bifida occulta of S-1 with ossicles.

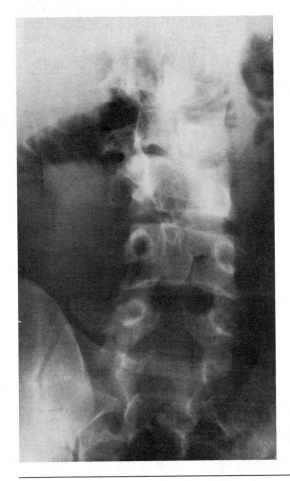

Multiple posterior arch defects with soft tissue mass. Spina bifida vera (manifesta).

continued

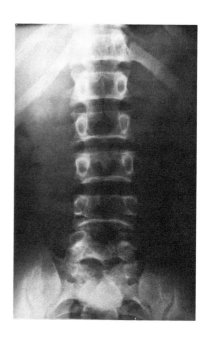

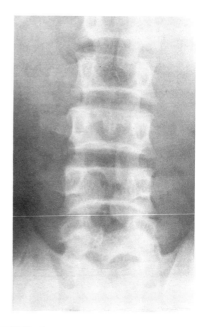

Two examples of multiple spina bifida occulta, no neurological manifestations.

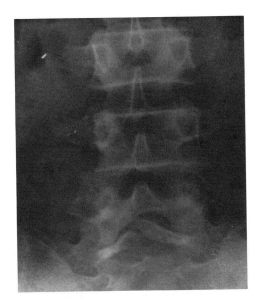

S-1 spina bifida occulta.

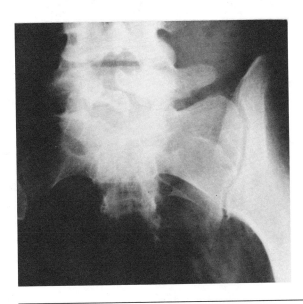

L-5 spina bifida occulta.

Knife Clasp Deformity

A knife clasp (clasped knife) deformity radiographically presents as a long spinous process of L-5 with a spina bifida occulta (posterior arch defect) of the first sacral segment. This long spinous process may be formed by fusion of the L-5 spinous process with the first sacral tubercle. Occasionally it has been associated with low back pain with radiculopathy, especially in hyperextension. This is possibly due to the L-5 spinous process impinging on the stump of the lamina of S-1 or on the fibrous membrane overlying the area of the spina bifida occulta, pressing on a nerve root or the cauda equina. When symptomatic, flexion exercises may be beneficial. Surgical removal or shortening of the spinous process has also been recorded as a successful therapy.

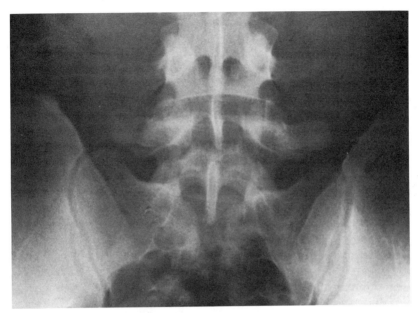

Knife clasp deformity. Bilateral L-5 spondylolysis (pars interarticularis defects) and asymmetrical facets at L-4–L-5.

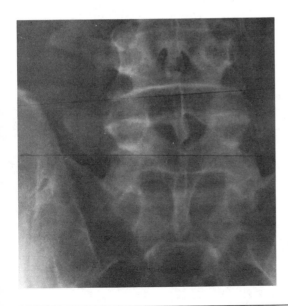

Knife clasp deformity. Long L-5 spinous process with S-1 posterior arch defect.

Transitional Segments

Variations in the number of segments in each spinal region occur in approximately 20% of skeletons, the total number of segments seldom varies. A vertebra at a transitional level may take on characteristics of both areas. This is most common at the lumbosacral and thoracolumbar junctions. If the transverse processes of the last lumbar segment are large, they will actually form true joints with a cartilaginous surface and articular capsules. Ligamentous articular connections are present and a bursa may also be present. When a lumbosacral transitional segment is present, the position of the weight bearing platform is usually altered. Sacralization (sometimes referred to as Bertolotti's syndrome) or lumbarization, shortens or lengthens the column. A short column is probably better fitted for heavy work, while a longer column has slightly increased mobility, and therefore is probably weakened. Considering that these conditions are congenital, the true clinical picture is relative to the muscular development and functional education. Unilateral or asymmetrical alterations result in asymmetrical mobility and strength of parts and may predispose the patient to musculoligamentous injuries. Transitional segments frequently have rudimentary articular processes. Bilateral and symmetrical manifestations are less common than asymmetrical findings. Sometimes the unilateral form is associated with scoliosis showing considerable rotation and torsion of the vertebral bodies.

Symptoms often appear initially after injury, illness, weight gain (such as pregnancy), unaccustomed activity, or working in an unusual or cramped position. Low back pain is the most common complaint, frequently localized at the lumbosacral region. It should be remembered that when a transitional segment is present it may not always be cause for low back complaint. Bilateral and symmetrical findings are more apt to be stable segments and may not be clinically significant.

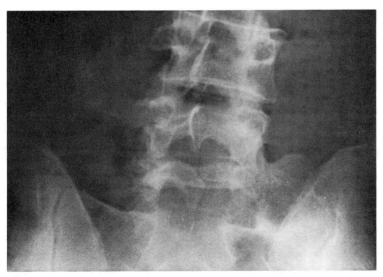

Unilateral transitional segment with mild sclerosis noted along articulation. Also noted facetal tropism between L-3–L-4, L-4–L-5, and spina bifida occulta of L-5 and S-1.

continued

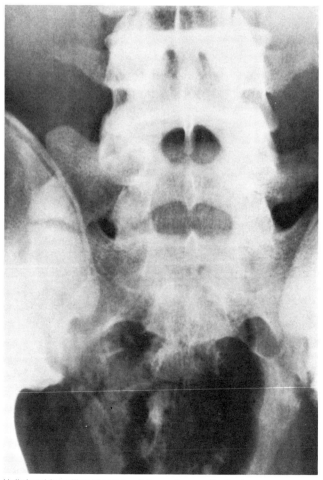
Unilateral transitional segment (pseudosacralization).

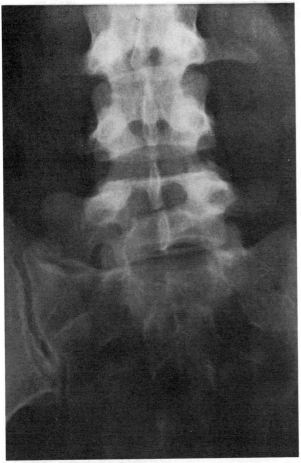

Unilateral transitional segment (pseudosacralization) with mild L-5 spina bifida occulta.

continued

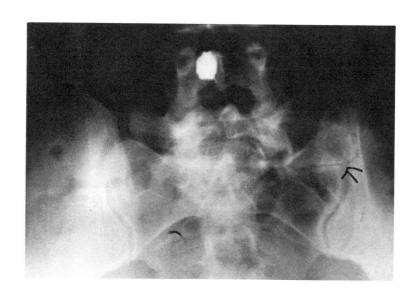

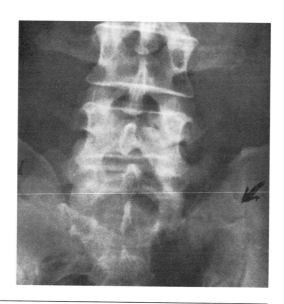

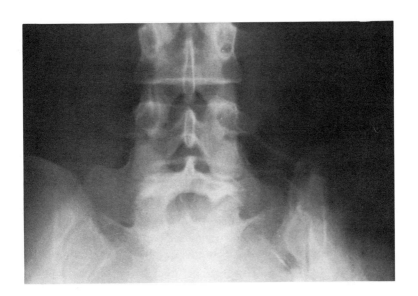

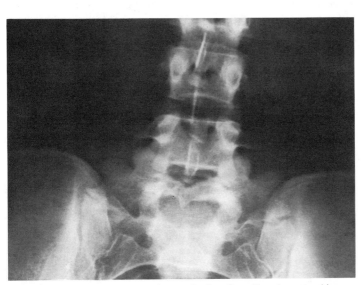

Four examples of bilateral pseudosacralization (transitional segments).

Transitional Segments

Hemivertebra

A hemivertebra is the failure or improper development of a portion of a vertebral body. Several different presentations of this are noted.

1. A single round or oval mass located between two vertebral bodies, as it matures it often coalesces with one or both of the vertebrae. In the thoracic spine, a pedicle and a rib process are usually associated
2. A wedge-shaped, triangular mass
3. Multiple portions of varying sizes and shapes
4. Multiple, with a unilateral bar failure of segmentation, may be accompanied by fusion and anomalies of ribs
5. Balanced—two or more hemivertebrae that compensate and negate significant spinal deformity. Their peak incidence is around the T-10 level

Marked angulation may simulate a fracture. Single or multiple hemivertebrae are a major cause of congenital scoliosis and kyphoscoliosis. Scoliosis occurs in 15% to 20% of cases however, if the findings are solitary, a wedge, or a balanced hemivertebra, they are usually not associated with rapid progression. This is true in approximately 50% of congenital deformities. Multiple hemivertebrae, however, on the same side, are often related to rapid progression of a curve.

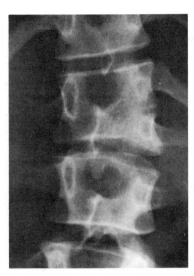
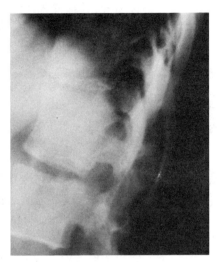

Two views of hemivertebra with two pedicles and one rib process.

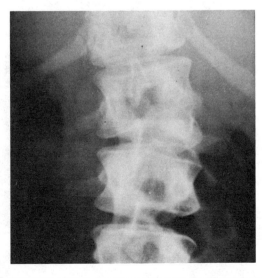

Hemivertebra. A somewhat ovoid mass that coalesced with the adjacent vertebra.

continued

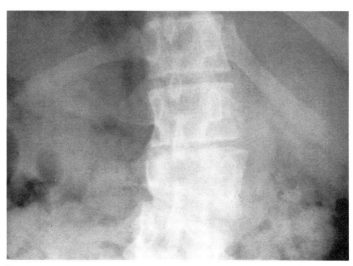

Unusual hemivertebra.

Hemivertebrae found at the lumbosacral junction pose a unique problem due to the lack of mobility below the anomaly. This results in a lateral shift of the trunk that may progress with growth.

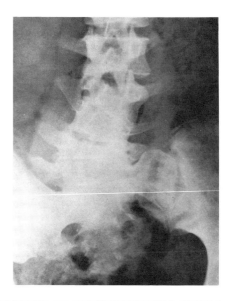

Butterfly Vertebra

Butterfly vertebrae are believed to develop due to the persistence of the notochord or a sagittal cleavage that extends through the vertebral body, sometimes called an anterior spina bifida. The vertebra above and below mold into the deficient centers of the affected vertebra. These anomalies have no clinical significance other than the biomechanical problems created.

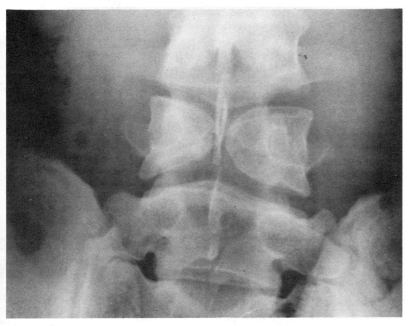

Butterfly vertebra. Also note transitional segment.

Failure of Segmentation

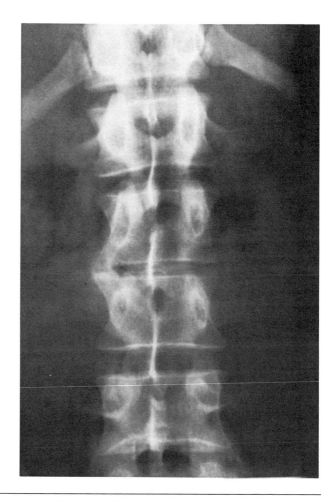

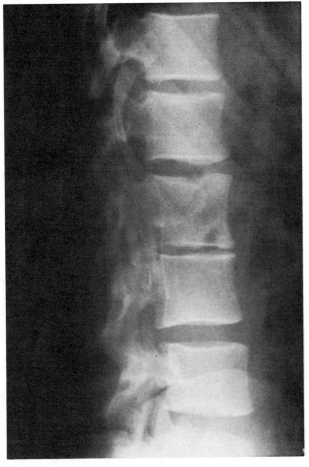

Two examples of failure of segmentation. Note bar connecting the two segments.

continued

Failure of Segmentation

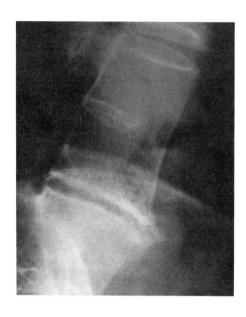

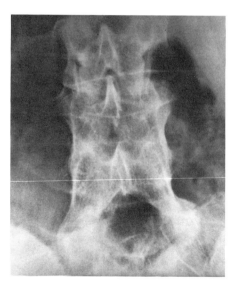

Two views of congenital block vertebra of L-4, L-5. Note the disc degeneration between L-5 and S-1.

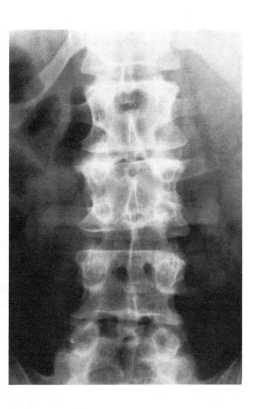

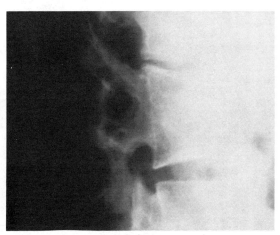

Two pictures of block vertebra. Note two sets of pedicles and transverse processes.

Failure of Segmentation

Anomalous Articulations

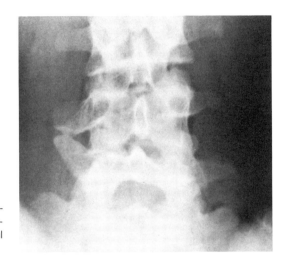

Anomalous articulation between the transverse processes of L-4–L-5. Lateral bending was restricted.

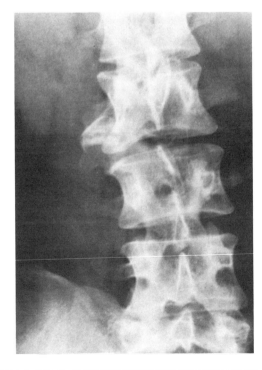

Anomalous articulation between the facets of L-3–L-4 with reactive sclerosis.

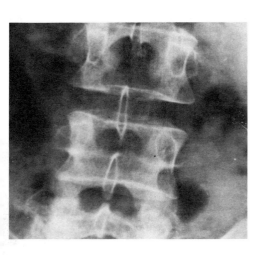

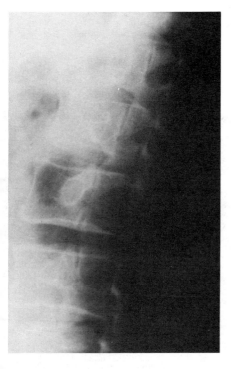

Two examples of accessory facet joint.

Anomalous Articulations

Asymmetrical Facets

This is a general cLAssification and may include alterations in size, orientation, and development. Tropism (which means a turning) is a subclassification of asymmetrical facets and is most descriptive when there are differences in orientation.

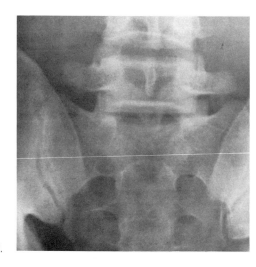

Facet tropism at L-4–L-5, L-5–S-1.

Tropism

The posterior elements allow and limit mobility, thus playing an important role in maintaining the stability of the spine. Clinical significance has been attributed to variations in the orientation of the articular processes, especially at the lumbosacral junction. Poorly developed or asymmetrically formed processes suggest mechanical instability and susceptibility to ligamentous injury. Arthritis tends to be more commonly associated with tropic facets. This may lead to lumbar instability manifesting itself as joint rotation which occurs toward the side of the more oblique facet. This may place additional stress on the annulus fibrosis of the intervertebral disc and capsular ligaments of the apophyseal joints. Studies by Farfan and Sullivan indicate that the incidence of annular tears is related to the orientation of the facets. They found that tropism leads to asymmetrical degeneration, often due to abnormal rotatory stress on the annulus. Protrusion will occur more often on the side of the more oblique joint surface. It should be remembered that asymptomatic annular tears are not uncommon and that each patient must individually be evaluated clinically and historically to determine the true relevance of this condition. Lutz suggests a different theory. The asymmetrical orientation of the articular facets develops during life because of unilateral stress and therefore cannot be considered a congenital disorder.

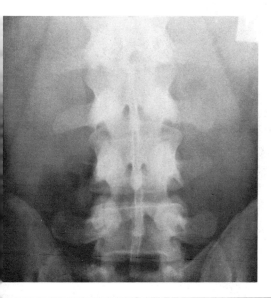

Tropism of articular facets between L-4–L-5, L-5–S-1. Spina bifida occulta of S-1.

Hypoplasia/Agenesis

Absence of lumbar or sacral articular processes is rare, and should not be confused with a destructive lesion. Deficiencies of articular processes in the lower spine are not at all uncommon. They do present with interesting compensatory features, e.g., unusual articulations between neural arches or hyperplasia of remaining structures. In the presence of these bony deficiencies, the ligamentation flavum and fibrous structures are unusually tough.

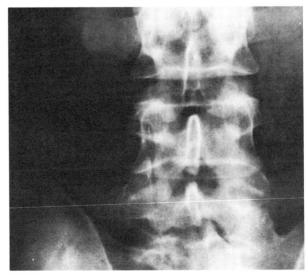

Hypoplasia of the L-5–S-1 articular facets with compensatory hyperplasia on the opposite side.

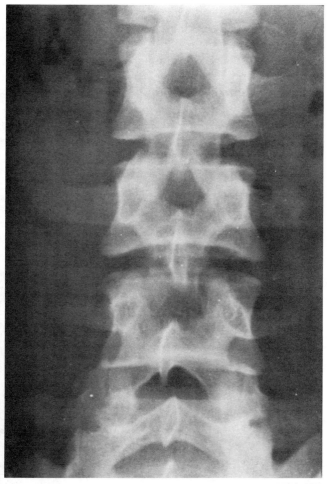

Hypoplastic inferior articular facets of the L-3 and asymmetry of the L-5–S-1 facets.

Persistent Secondary Ossification Centers

Persistent secondary ossification centers are determined when a small, triangular bony ossicle is found at the tip of the inferior articular process of a vertebra. They have joint surfaces and are covered with cartilage. Usually encountered in the lumbar region around the L-3 level they are more common in males. The ossicle has been called the ossicle of Oppenheimer. Oppenheimer has stated that each spinal articular process may have three to four separate centers of ossification. A much less frequent finding is the persistent apophysis of the superior articular facet. These may be confused with a fracture. An isolated fracture of this process, however, is very unlikely, without the neural arch or body also being involved. If a fracture does occur, it would be the result of a severe trauma of a rotary character, usually with the spine flexed. The fracture would produce marked pain and localized tenderness. These can often be differentiated by the roundness of their continuous marginal outlines. Most feel that the persistent apophysis is of no clinical significance. Others have stated that these are usually asymptomatic unless they become wedged in the apophyseal joint space.

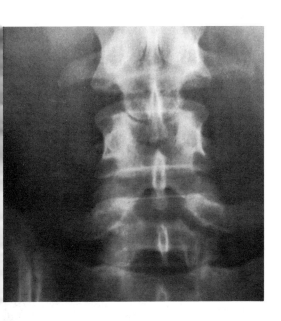

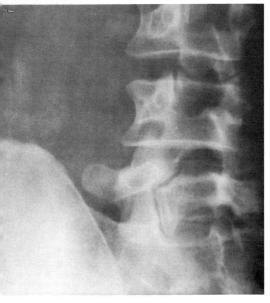

Bilateral persistent apophyses (secondary center of ossification) of the inferior articular facets of L-3. Also noted are the wide pars interarticularis defect (spondylolysis) of L-5 (two views).

Limbus Bone

The limbus bone is a small, triangular bony ossicle often adjacent to the anterior aspect of the lumbar vertebral bodies, more often seen at the superior aspect. A number of theories are proposed as to the origin of this. It may represent a persistent secondary ossification center or be the result of marginal disc herniation prior to the fusion of the ring epiphysis. It may also be the result of an anterior herniation of discal material, in which case irregularity of the anterior surfaces is often present and discography usually demonstrates the migration of disc material.

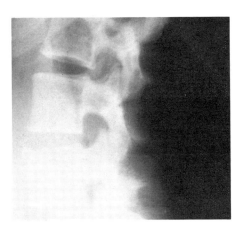

Limbus bones adjacent to antero-superior aspect of L-5.

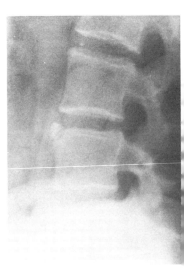

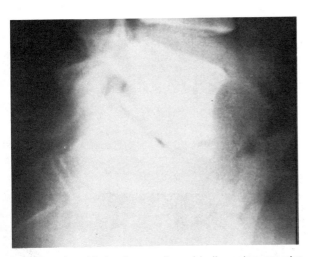

Two examples of limbus bone adjacent to the antero-superior aspect of the L-4 vertebral body.

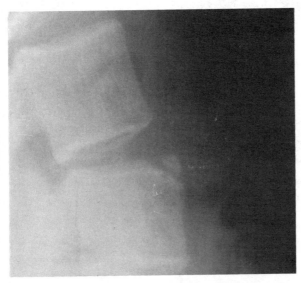

Limbus bone adjacent to the antero-inferior aspect of L-5. Note the vacuum phenomenon in L-5–S-1 disc space.

Nuclear Impressions

Nuclear impressions are endplate depressions (invaginations) secondary to notochordal remnants. They should be differentiated from Schmorl's nodes. They are usually broader, often smoother, and more commonly posterior manifestations. These are not clinically significant.

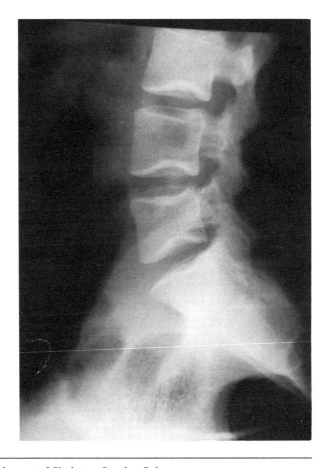

Iliolumbar Ligament Calcification

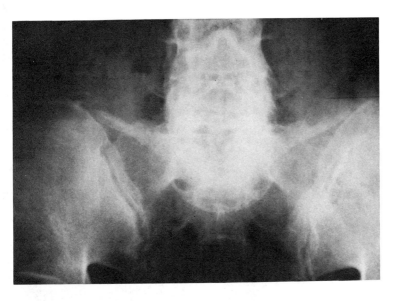

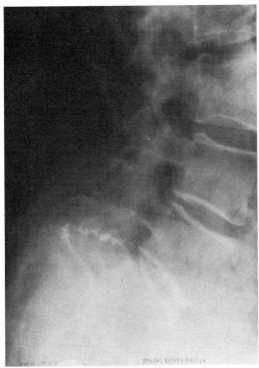

Iliolumbar ligament calcification is probably the body's response to establish stability and support an unusual weakened area. Note grade IV spondylolisthesis (two views).

Pelvis

Paraglenoid Fossae
Os Acetabuli
Persistent Growth Centers
Ligament Calcification
Phleboliths

Paraglenoid Fossae

Paraglenoid fossae (preauricular sulci) are crescent-shaped defects of varying sizes just lateral to the inferior aspect of the sacroiliac joints on the ilium. They are usually bilateral but not necessarily symmetrical. This finding is most frequently encountered in females. The groove of paraglenoid fossae transmits the superior branch of the gluteal artery and supplies insertion for a portion of the sacroiliac ligament. Some researchers feel that the reason this is more commonly encountered in the multiparous female is related to the stress on the ligament during the birthing process.

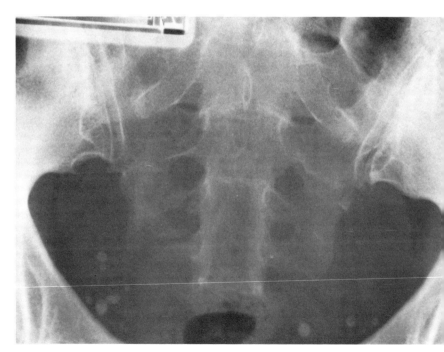

Bilateral asymmetrical paraglenoid fossae—and numerous phleboliths are evident. Also noted is anomalous formation of the sacral foramen.

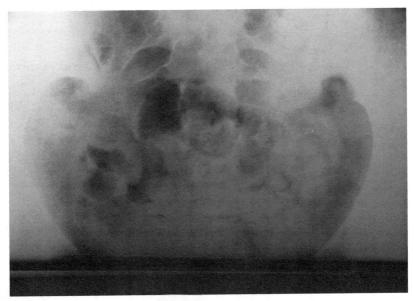
Bilateral asymmetrical paraglenoid fossae.

Os Acetabuli

Os acetabuli are round or oval ossicles of varying sizes adjacent to the upper rim of the acetabulum. This is felt to be an ununited growth center or a sesamoid bone, without clinical significance.

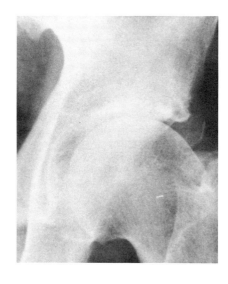

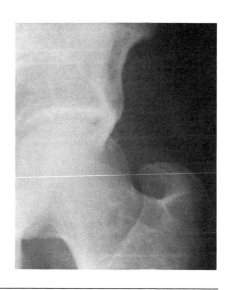

Persistent Growth Centers

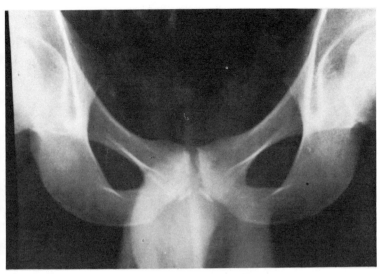

Persistent apophyses of the pubic bones.

Ligament Calcification

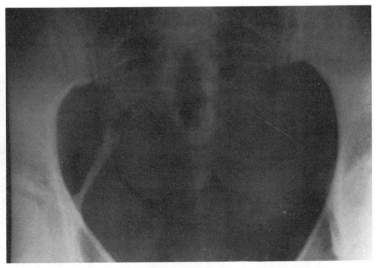

Ligamentous calcification or ossification is usually of no clinical significance.

Phleboliths

Phleboliths are the most common pelvic calcification and are round or structureless, measuring 2 to 5 mm in diameter. The number may vary from one to multiple. They are frequent around the valves of the veins, and normally of no clinical significance.

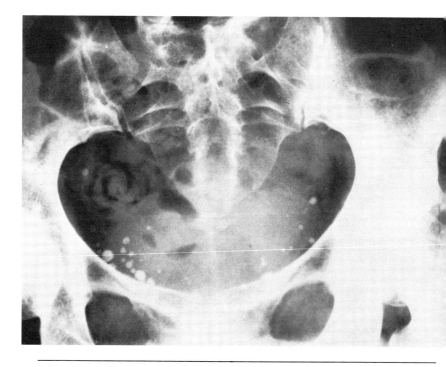

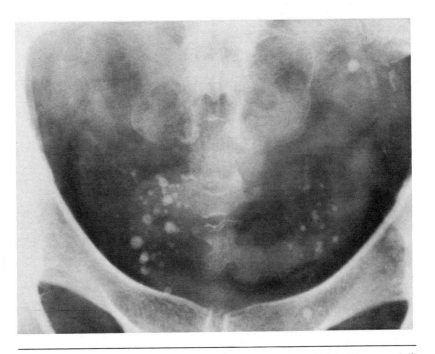

Upper Extremity

Radioulnar Synostosis
Conoid Process
Supracondylar Process
Persistent Growth Center

Radioulnar Synostosis

Radioulnar synostosis is a union of the proximal radius and ulna. It is equal in distribution between males and females and is bilateral in approximately 60% of patients. Clinically, loss of rotation of the forearm is present. This often goes unnoticed because the individual compensates by rotation of the shoulder.

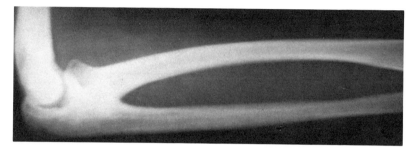

Conoid Process

The conoid process (tubercle) is a bony cone-shaped eminence of variable size on the under-surface of the clavicle. It serves as the attachment for the conoid ligament. It may, on occasion, form an anomalous articulation with the coracoid process. Generally, it is not clinically significant.

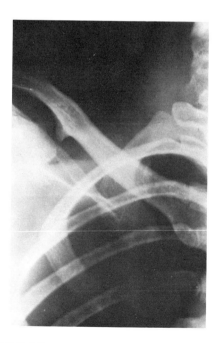

Supracondylar Process

The supracondylar process arises from the anteromedial aspect of the distal portion of the diaphysis of the humerus. It represents a prominent attachment of the pronator teres muscle. It is directed distally, different from an osteochondroma which is directed away from the joint. These are typically without symptoms, but fractures have been recorded.

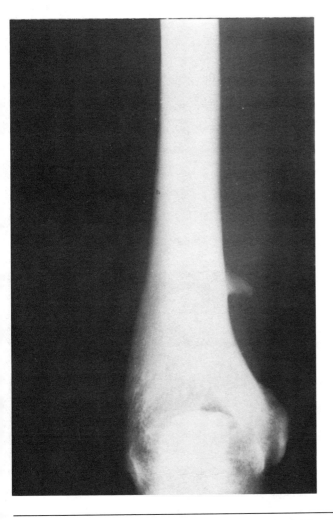

Persistent Growth Center

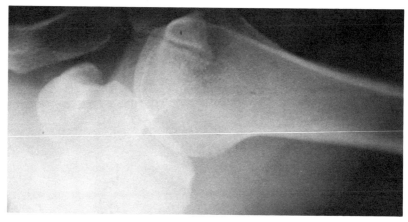

Persistent apophysis of the acromion process.

Lower Extremity

Fabella
Os Trigonum
Bipartite Patella

Fabella

The fabella ("little bean") is a sesamoid bone frequently found in the tendon of the lateral head of the gastrocnemius muscle. Variations in size, shape, and number have been noted. This is rarely visible before 12 years of age and is frequently bilateral. Radiographically, these are best visualized on a lateral knee film in the posterior soft tissues. It has been reported that a fabella may become enlarged and roughened in cases where degenerative disease is present, however, they are not felt to be clinically significant.

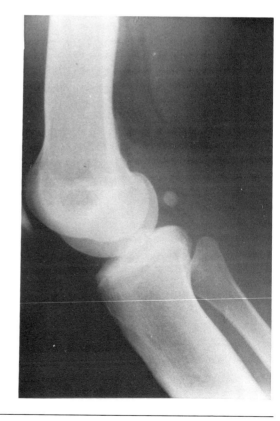

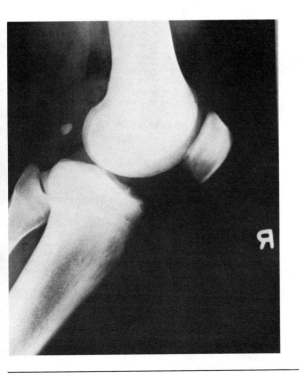

Os Trigonum

Os trigonum (talus secundarius) is a separate ossification center at the posterior aspect of the talus to which the talofibular ligament is attached. Its shape varies from a small, triangular fragment to one or more rounded or oval ossicles. The division from the talus may be incomplete. This finding has been reported as occurring in about 10% of all individuals and is of no clinical significance.

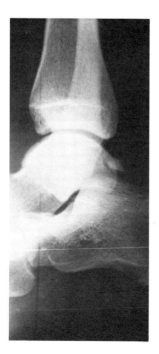
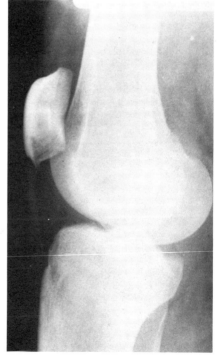

Bipartite Patella

Bipartite (or multipartite) patella may be divided into two or more fragments. Usually the smaller fragments are located at its superolateral aspect. This finding is usually bilateral in approximately 80% of patients. It is not considered clinically significant and should not be mistaken for a fracture.

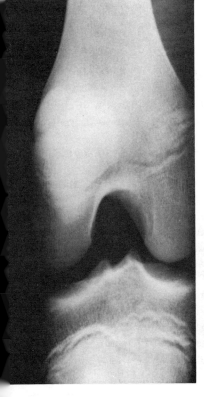
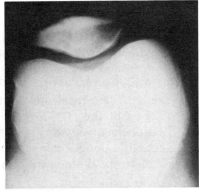

BIBLIOGRAPHY

Applbaum GY, Byrk D: Elongation of the anterior tubercle of a cervical vertebral transverse process: An unusual variant Skeletal Radiology 10:267, 1983.

Arcomano JP, Karas, Spyros: Congenital absence of the lumbosacral articular processes. Skeletal Radiology 133–134 1982.

Barrows EH: Clinical relevance of radiological abnormalities o the craniovertebral junction. British Journal of Radiolog 54:195–202, 1981.

Barson AJ: Spina bifida: The significance of the level and exten of the defect to the morphogenesis. Developmental Medicine Child Neurology 12(2):129–144, 1970.

Boone D, Parsons D, Lachmann SM, Sherwood T: Spina bifid. occulta: Lesion or anomaly. Clinical Radiology 36(2):159–161 1985.

Castellvi AE, Goldstein LA, Chan DAK: Lumbosacral transitional vertebrae and their relationship with lumbar extradura defects. Spine 9(5):493–495, 1984.

Christenson PC: The radiologic study of the normal spine Radiologic Clinic of North America 15(2):133–154, 1977.

Cyron BM, Hutton WC: Articular tropism and stability of th lumbar spine. Spine 5(2):168–172, 1980.

D'Ambrosia RD: The neck. The back—thoracic and lumba spine. In Musculoskeletal Disorders. Philadelphia, JB Lippincott, 1977.

Dawson EG, Smith L: Atlantoaxial subluxation in children du to vertebral anomalies. Journal of Bone and Joint Surger 582–587, 1979.

Dolan KD: Cervicobasilar relationships. Radiologic Clinics o North America 15(2): 155–166, 1977.

Etter M, Lewis E: Osseous abnormalities of the thoracic cag seen in forty thousand consecutive chest photoroentgeno grams. American Journal Roentgenologic and Radiatio Therapy 51(5):593–599, 1944.

Feldman F: The symptomatic spine: Relevant and irrelevar roentgen variants and variations. Orthopedic Clinics of Nort America 14(1):119–145, 1983.

Feldman F: Miscellaneous localized conditions: A whirlwind re view of the "Oh My Aching Back" syndrome. Seminars i Roentgenology XIV:58–75, 1979.

Fixsen J: Congenital abnormalities of the limbs. British Journa of Hospital Medicine 26(3):193, 1981.

Fraser RG, Pare P: Seventeen diseases of the diaphragm and chest wall. In Diagnosis of Diseases of the Chest. Philadelphia, WB Saunders, 1978.

Gillespie HW: The significance of congenital lumbosacral abnormalities. British Journal of Radiology 12(257): 270–275, 1949.

Gooban JE, Erickson F, Pate D, Sartoris DJ, Resnick D: Symptomatic clasp-knife deformity of the spinous process (to be published in Spine).

Greenfield GB: Radiology of Bone Diseases. Philadelphia, JB Lippincott, 1969.

Guebert GM, Thompson JR: Radiology case report: Os odontoideum. ACA Journal of Chiropractic 20(9): 69–71, 1986.

Gwinn JL, Smith JL: Acquired and congenital absence of the odontoid process. From Departments of Radiology of the Children's Hospital, Los Angeles and the University of Southern California School of Medicine 88(3): 224–431, 1962.

Hadley LA: Disturbances of development. Disturbances of cervical spine development. Observation of the lumbosacral level. In Anatomico-Roentgenographic Studies of the Spine, 4th ed, 1964.

Hensinger RN, Lang LE, MacErven GD: Klippel-Feil syndrome. Journal of Bone and Joint Surgery 56(6):1246–1253, 1974.

Hensinger RN: Osseous anomalies of the craniovertebral junction. Spine 11(4): 323–333, 1986.

Jackson R: Etiology—Anomalies. In The Cervical Syndrome. Springfield, Ill., Thomas, 4th ed, 1977.

Keats TE: An Atlas of Normal Roentgen Variants That May Simulate Disease. Chicago, Yearbook, 1984.

Leatherman KD, Diskson RA: Two stage corrective surgery for congenital deformities of the spine. Journal of Bone and Joint Surgery 61(3): 324–328, 1979.

Magora A, Schwartz A: Relation between the low back pain syndrome and x-ray findings. Scandinavian Journal of Rehabilitative Medicine 10(3):135–145, 1978.

Maurer EL: Biomechanical considerations. In Practical Applied Roentgenology. Baltimore, Williams and Wilkins, 1983.

McRae DL: The significance of abnormalities of the cervical spine. American Journal of Roentgenology Radium Therapy and Nuclear Medicine 84(1): 3–25, 1960.

Meschan I: Congenital and hereditary abnormalities of the skeletal system. In Analysis of Roentgen Signs in General Radiology. Philadelphia, WB Saunders, 1973.

Mitchell GA: The significance of lumbosacral transitional vertebrae. British Journal of Surgery, 147–157.

Murray RO, Jacobson HG: Congenital disorders. In The Radiology of Skeletal Disorders. New York, WB Saunders, 1977.

Nasca RJ, Stilling FH, Stell HH: Progression of congenital scoliosis due to hemivertebrae with bars. Journal of Bone and Joint Surgery 57(4): 456–466, 1975.

Ogden JA, Conlogue GJ, Phillips MS, Bronson ML: Sprengel's deformity. Skeletal Radiology 4:204–211, 1979.

Paul LW, Juhl JH: Miscellaneous skeletal anomalies and syndromes. In The Essentials of Roentgen Interpretation. Maryland, Harper and Row, 1972.

Reeder MM, Felson B: Gamuts in Radiology. Cincinnati, Audiovisual Radiology of Cincinnati, Inc, 1975.

Resnick D, Niwayama G: Normal anatomic variants and artifacts that may simulate disease (Keats). In Diagnosis of Bone and Joint Disorders. Philadelphia, WB Saunders, 1981.

Rothman RH, Simeone FA: Congenital skeletal anomalies. In The Spine. Philadelphia, WB Saunders, 1981.

Schmorl G, Junghanus H: Variations and malformations of the spine. Transitional regions of the spine. In The Human Spine in Health and Disease. New York, Grune and Stratton, 1971.

Slabaugh PB, Winter RB, Lonstein JE, Moe JH: Lumbosacral hemivertebrae. Spine 5(3):234–244, 1980.

Stark WA: Spina bifida occulta and engagement of the fifth lumbar spinous process. Clinical Orthopedics and Related Research 71–72, 1971.

Sutton D: Congenital skeletal anomalies. In Textbook of Radiology. New York, Longman, Inc, 1978.

Sycamore LK: Common congenital anomalies of the bony thorax. 51(5):593–599, 1944.

Wigh RE: The thoracolumbar and lumbosacral transitional junctions. Spine 5(3):215–222, 1980.

Wigh RE: The transitional lumbosacral osseous complex. Skeletal Radiology 8:127–131, 1981.

Wilk S, Zimmer EA: Borderlands in Normal and Early Pathology in Skeletal Roentgenology. New York, Grune and Stratton, 1968.

Wilkinson RH, Strand RD: Congenital anomalies and normal variants. Seminars in Roentgenology 14(1):7–19, 1979.

Willis TA: An analysis of vertebral anomalies. American Journal of Surgery 163–168, 1929.

Wright JA: Radiological refresher: Congenital and developmental abnormalities of the vertebrae. Journal of Small Animal Practice 625–634, 1979.

Glossary

Agenesis. Absence of a portion or all of a structure. However, many times in reference to a bony process it refers to failure of ossification, therefore not being depicted as an osseous structure.

Anode heel effect. X-rays emitting from the focal spot of the tube are less intense toward the anode and more intense away from it, (e.g., on an AP thoracic view the anode is placed toward the head). A more even penetration is achieved due to less thickness toward the head.

Anomaly. Deviation from normal standard, especially as a result of congenital or hereditary defects.

Anterior. Front. Term used when referring to the belly surface of the body.

Apophysis. An "offshoot." An outgrowth that adds width to the host bone, forms a process, tuberosity tubercle, for muscular or ligamentous attachment.

Artifact. Any foreign artificial product. A structure or substance not normally present, produced by some external agency or action.

Asymmetry (asymmetrical). Dissimilarity in corresponding parts on opposite sides of the body which are normally alike.

Basilar invagination (impression). Apparent indentation of the floor of the skull by the upper cervical spine, this may be a developmental anomaly or caused by abnormal softening of the bones. One method for determining this is to use McGregor's line. On a lateral cervical film, draw a line from the upper surface of the posterior margin of the hard palate to the most inferior part of the floor of the posterior fossa. Normally the tip of the odontoid does not project more than 4.5 mm above this line.

Canthomeatal line. A line from the outer corner of the eye (canthus) to the opening (meatus) of the ear.

Caudad (caudal). Toward the feet.

Cephalad. Toward the head.

Concavity. Hollowed out area. Rounded, somewhat depressed surface.

Congenital. Existing at and usually before birth, not hereditary.

Convexity. Rounded, somewhat elevated area.

Coronal. Passing through the body at a right angle to the median plane.

Correction factor. A number allowed for use of the Supertech; this corrects for variations in X-ray machines and for alterations from what was considered standard for the Supertech such as, 12:1, Bucky/Grid 40″ FFD.

Dorsal. Pertaining to the back.

Dysplasia. Abnormality in development. In pathology, an alteration in size, shape, and organization of adult cells.

Ectopic. Located away from normal position.

Epiphysis. The end of long bones or margins of flat bones adding length to the bone.

Extension. Movement by which two ends of any jointed part are drawn away from each other.

FFD. Film focal distance, distance usually measured in inches between the focal spot of the X-ray tube to the film.

Flexion. The act of bending or conditions of being bent.

Glabella. A smooth area on the frontal bone midway between the supraorbital ridges.

Grid. A grating used to reduce the amount of scatter radiation reaching the film, comprised of closely spaced narrow lead strips.

Horizontal. Parallel to the horizon (apparent intersection of the earth and sky as seen by an observer).

Hyperplasia. Abnormal multiplication or increase in the number of normal cells in normal arrangement in a tissue.

Hypoplasia. Incomplete or under development.

Kilovolt peak (kVp). Parameter that deals with contrast (black and white) on film.

Linear. Pertaining to or resembling a line. Straight.

Manifesta. True or obvious to the eye.

mAs. Milliampere second, primarily responsible for density on film.

Occulta. Hidden or concealed.

Palmar. Palm surface of the hand.

Prone. Lying face downward.

Posterior. Back or dorsal surface of the body.

Parallel. Being an equal distance apart at every point, two or more straight lines that do not intersect.

Perpendicular. Intersecting at or forming right angles.

Pseudoarthrosis. "False joint."

Recumbent. Lying down, reclining.

Rotate. Turn around on an axis, to twist.

Rudimentary. Imperfectly developed (vestigial).

Sagittal. A vertical plane extending from A to P, and separating left from right, parallel to median plane of the body.

SID. Source image distance = FFD distance for X-ray tube to film.

Supine. Lying with face or ventral surface up.

Supertech. A technique computer somewhat similar to a slide rule that helps the operator to determine proper parameters needed to produce a diagnostic film. It considers patient size, grids, screens, distance, age, alterations in density such as in osteopenia, atrophy, heavy musculature. It will provide variable kVp and mAs combinations.

Submental. Situated below the chin.

Vertical. Relating to the vertex (top); perpendicular to the horizon.

Ventral. Anterior or front belly.

Vera. True, obvious.

Index

Agenesis, 262–263, 292, 342–343
Anode heel effect, 28, 32, 36
Anomalous articulations, 270–271, 338, 339, 360
Anterior inferior iliac spine, 71
Anterior tubercle, 11, 19, 264, 274–275
Aortic knob, 229
Apophysis persistent (ununited), 259, 306, 344, 355, 362
Arch, 11, 211, 244, 258, 277, 316, 319, 322, 323
Arcuate foramen (foramen arcuale), 9, 276
Articular facets, 5, 11, 19, 34, 35, 43, 47, 51, 58, 341, 342, 343, 344, 345
Asymmetrical facets, 323, 340, 342
Atlas, 248, 272, 276, 282
  arch, 11, 211
  assimilation, 269
  cleft, 257, 259, 316
  hypertrophy of anterior tubercle, 264
  hypoplasia of posterior tubercle, 262
  posterior tubercle, 207, 271
Azygos lobe, 312

Bertolotti's syndrome, 324
Bifid
  rib, 294
  spinous process, 5
Bipartite, 367
Block vertebrae, 244–251, 252–253, 336–337
Bowel, 78, 80, 84, 86, 88
Breathing, 28, 36, 219, 226, 230, 234, 252, 291
Bursa, 270, 324
Butterfly vertebrae, 333

Calcifications
  costal cartilage, 280, 295–298
  iliolumbar ligament, 349
  nuchal ligament, 278–279
  physiological, 280–281
  pineal gland, 280, 281
  railroad track, 281, 295, 296
  styloid, 282–283
  thyroid cartilage, 280, 281
  wagging tongue, 295, 296
Canthomeatal, 196, 200, 204, 208, 214
Carpal synostosis, 166, 178
Cervical rib, 274, 284–287, 294
Clinoid
  anterior, 207
  posterior, 207
Condyle, 95, 99, 103, 106, 211, 264, 272
Conoid process, 360
Coracoid, 138, 140–141, 142, 360
Coronoid process, 147, 151, 155

Costophrenic recess, 229
Costotranverse articulation, 31, 229
Costovertebral articulation, 31

Dens, 11, 19, 264
Diaphragm, 28, 31, 219, 226, 229, 230, 233, 234, 291

Ectopic, 292
Epicondyle, 95, 103, 147, 151, 158
External auditory meatus, 207, 232

Fabella, 364–365
Facet, 57
   accessory, 339
   asymmetry, 323, 340, 342
   hyperplastic, 342, 343
   hypoplastic, 342
   ossicle of Oppenheimer, 344
   persistent secondary growth center, 344–345, 346
   tropism, 324, 340, 341
Failure of segmentation, 244–251, 252–253, 269, 334–336
Fibrous band, 284, 291, 316
Forked rib, 294
Foramen, 352
   intervertebral, 19, 47, 58, 233, 244, 246, 252
   magnum, 203, 207, 269
   sacral, 43, 352
Fossae
   antecubital, 144, 148
   glenoid, 140, 141
   intercondylar, 95, 103, 106
   paraglenoid, 352–353
   popliteal, 72
   rhomboid, 300

Gonad shield, 52

Hahn's fissures, 304

Hemivertebra, 252, 256, 328–331
   dorsal, 307
   unbalanced, 305
Hyperplasia (hyperplastic), 285, 342
Hypoplasia (hypoplastic), 252, 262—263, 342—343

Identification, 182
Iliopectineal line, 66
Intercalary bones, 273
Interosseous membrane, 95
Intertrochanteric crest, 66, 71
Intrathoracic ribs, 291
Ischial tuberosity, 71, 75

Klippel-Feil syndrome, 252–253, 254
Knife clasp deformity, 322–323

Lamina, 11, 43, 51, 55, 316, 322
Lateral mass, 7
Limbus bone, 346–347
Lumbarization, 324

Malleolus, 108, 109, 110, 111, 112, 114, 119
Medial ends, 301
Mediastinal clear space, 233
Mortise view, 110
Multipartite, 367

Nasal turbinate, 199
Nuchal bones, 278–279
Nuclear impression, 348

Occipitalization, 248, 269
Odontoid process, 7, 211, 264–265, 268, 269, 271
Olecranon process, 147, 151, 155, 156, 158
Omovertebral bone, 254, 255
Orbit, 199, 207, 211

Os acetabuli, 354
  odontoidium, 264–267
  trigonum, 366
Ossicle of Oppenheimer, 344
Ossiculum terminale, 264, 268
Osteophyte, 244, 274

Paraglenoid fossa, 352—353
Paramastoid processes, 271, 272
Paracondylar processes, 272
Pars interarticularis, 51, 323, 345
Patella, 90, 92, 95, 99, 100, 103–106, 367
Pectus
  excavatum, 310
  carinatum, 311
Pedicle, 11, 19, 31, 43, 51, 55, 261, 337
Pillar view, 20–23
Phleboliths, 352, 356–357
Plateau (tibial), 95, 103
Ponticle
  posterior, 276–277
Proatlas, 264
Process
  supracondylar, 361
  conoid, 360
Pseudoarthrosis, 290
Pseudosacralization, 326, 327

Radioulnar synostosis, 360
Ribs
  bifid, 294
  cervical, 274, 284–285
  ectopic, 292
  forked, 294
  intrathoracic, 291
Rhomboid, 300

Sacralization, 324
Sandbags, 8, 64, 68
Schmorl's nodes, 348
Scoliosis, 32, 36, 44, 59–61, 244, 252, 305, 324
Sella turcica, 207, 208
Secondary centers of ossification, 344–345, 346

Spina bifida occulta, 252, 257–260, 305, 316–321, 322, 325, 327, 341
  cervical spine, 257–259
  lumbar spine, 316–321, 327
  thoracic spine, 260
Spina bifida vera, 316, 319
Spondylolisthesis, 316
Spondylolysis, 316, 323, 345, 349
Sprengel's deformity, 252, 254–255
Stress views, 142
Styloid process, 282–283
  radial, 169, 176–177
  ulnar, 169, 176–177, 185, 189
Sunrise (tangential), 104—106
Supertech, 196, 200, 204, 208, 216, 219
Supracondylar process, 361
Suprascapular process, 254
Synostosis, 269, 293, 360
Swimmer's view, 24

Tangential (sunrise), 104–106
Transitional segments, 324–327, 333
Tropism, 324–325, 340, 341
Tubercle
  anterior, 11, 19, 264, 274–275
  posterior, 11, 19, 262, 270, 360
  radial, 147, 151
  sacral, 43, 322
Tuberosity
  greater, 140
  ischial, 66, 71, 75
  lesser, 141
  tibial, 95, 99

Uncinate process, 5
Uncovertebral joint, 244

Vertebra
  block, 244–251, 252–253
  butterfly, 333
  Hemi, 252, 256, 305, 307, 328, 331

Wasp waist, 244, 245